KU-616-426

South Dublin Libraries
www.southdublinlibraries.ie

The Imperfect Nutritionist

7 Principles of Healthy Eating

JENNIFER MEDHURST

The Imperfect Nutritionist

7 Principles of Healthy Eating

For anyone who is struggling and trying to do better.

Text copyright 2023 © Jennifer Medhurst

Design and layout copyright 2023
© Octopus Publishing Group Limited

Photography copyright 2023 © Nick Hopper

Publishing Director: Judith Hannam

Publisher: Joanna Copestick

Editor: Vicky Orchard

Editorial Assistant: Emma Hanson

Design: Imagist

Photography: Nick Hopper

Props & food styling: Vanessa Lewis

Proofreading: Vicki Murrell

Production: Katherine Hockley

An Hachette UK Company
www.hachette.co.uk

First published in Great Britain
in 2023 by Kyle Books, an imprint of
Octopus Publishing Group Limited
Carmelite House
50 Victoria Embankment
London EC4Y 0DZ
www.kylebooks.co.uk

ISBN: 9781914239755

Distributed in the US by Hachette Book Group,
1290 Avenue of the Americas, 4th and 5th Floors,
New York, NY 10104

Distributed in Canada by Canadian Manda Group,
664 Annette St., Toronto, Ontario, Canada M6S 2C8

Jennifer Medhurst is hereby identified as the author
of this work in accordance with section 77 of the
Copyright, Designs and Patents Act 1988.

All rights reserved. No part of this work may be reproduced
or utilised in any form or by any means, electronic or
mechanical, including photocopying, recording or by
any information storage and retrieval system, without
the prior written permission of the publisher.

Printed and bound in China

10 9 8 7 6 5 4 3 2 1

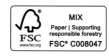

The information in this book is not intended to replace
or conflict with the advice given to you by your doctor
or other health professionals. All matters regarding
your health should be discussed with your doctor or
other health professional. The author and publisher
disclaim any liability directly or indirectly from the
use of the material in this book by any person.

The information in this book is correct at the time
of going to print.

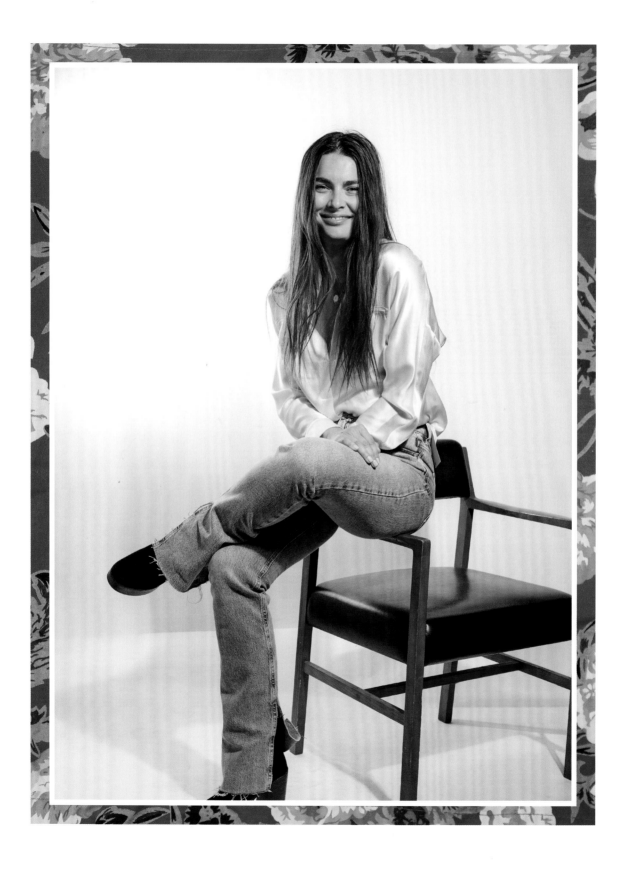

There was a time when I thought the food we ate had little or no relationship to our health. I worked a 50-hour week, ate out several nights a week, and on the others had a microwaveable meal. I had no energy, yet struggled to sleep or relax. I wanted to be better but didn't think I had the time to become one of those 'healthy people'.

Fast forward a few years, a degree, and many nutrition courses later, and my life has changed dramatically. After my first few years practising as a nutritionist, I started to notice that no matter what aspect of a client's health I was dealing with, there were some common principles which underpinned any nutrition plan I was writing – ultimate truths if you will. I started to think, what if these principles could be grouped together to form the foundation of any healthy diet? What if they weren't dependent on the latest fad but centred on clear, evidence-based guidance that anyone can apply to their everyday life in an easy and accessible way?

The principles are:

Focus on whole foods

Be diverse

What the fat!?

Include fermented, prebiotic and probiotic foods

Reduce refined carbohydrates

Be aware of liquids

Eat mindfully

Quite often prospective clients are concerned that if they come to see a nutritionist, they will be stuck on a boring diet of salad leaves or must go vegan. This misperception of what healthy actually looks like is why I felt compelled to create The Imperfect Nutritionist. I'm not an aggressively strict clinician who does everything perfectly, nor am I a laissez-faire foodie. I'm a normal person, who eats everything, makes mistakes and wants to live my life but be healthy while doing it. So what if you can't make the perfect buckwheat flour pancakes, and you don't know what an açai bowl is,

but you're not a junk-food lover either? Who was talking to these people in the middle? The people that want to live their lives but be healthy while doing it. That's where The Imperfect Nutritionist comes in. This is not a massive diet overhaul; these are simple principles which are ultimate truths. They are not sexy or glamorous, but are the established scientific principles that underpin any healthy diet and they aren't going anywhere. I hope to empower people with accurate information they can then take and apply to their own lives, according to their own unique likes, dislikes, tastes or cultural preferences. To live the life they want to.

For too long the diet industry had a 'one size fits all' restrictive approach, 'avoid carbs', 'fats are bad', 'no gluten'. This, combined with an overwhelming volume of conflicting information, means that people often struggle to sustain a diet or don't know what they should be doing so give up on the idea of 'being healthy' entirely. I wanted to create a simple approach that embraced each person's own uniqueness. One that empowers people with accessible accurate information to easily create a sustainable and enjoyable way of eating, according to their individual tastes. This isn't about what you should exclude, but what you can include. You love pizza and ice cream? Great let's keep them in your diet. But what else can we add in? This positive inclusive approach makes for a sustainable way of eating, and consequently one that has a far greater chance of being successful in the long term.

This book is about more not about less. It's meant to be easy and fun, to tantalize and inspire. I look forward to going on your health journey with you...

Jennifer

Getting Started: Ingredient List

I always aim to have my kitchen stocked up with healthy ingredients. Below is by no means an exhaustive list but it's a good place to start.

Grains

Brown rice

Pasta (my preference is for brown rice pasta, but any kind is fine so long as it is high quality and as unprocessed as possible)

Quinoa (other grains worth trying are buckwheat, bulgur wheat, amaranth, pearl barley, spelt, polenta and millet)

Rice cakes or oatcakes

Good quality bread (opt for brown rather than white, regular or gluten-free, depending on your preference; sourdough is also a good option)

Whole rolled oats (regular or gluten free depending on your preference)

Beans and legumes

There's a huge range of beans and legumes from lentils to black beans and chickpeas, so take your pick! Buying dried versions, then soaking and cooking them is the best (and cheapest) option but is time-consuming, so canned is usually more convenient. The manufacturing process can differ – some beans and legumes are cooked and then canned, others are cooked in the can, which means they can be harder to digest. The higher quality the brand, the more likely it is they will have been cooked first.

Condiments

Tahini

Soy sauce or tamari (a gluten-free fermented soy sauce)

Apple cider vinegar (raw with the mother), red wine vinegar, sherry vinegar, balsamic vinegar

Dijon mustard, wholegrain mustard (look for sugar-free varieties made with apple cider vinegar)

Herbs and spices

Mixed herbs, herbs de Provence, chilli flakes, cumin, turmeric

Salt and pepper (of course)

Cinnamon, nutmeg, fresh vanilla pods, vanilla essence

Oils and fats

Extra virgin olive oil is hands down the winning oil. It's loaded with beneficial plant chemicals and several studies show it has wide-ranging health benefits. Make sure you're getting the minimally processed stuff by looking out for the LOT number and harvest date on the bottle.

Nuts and seeds

Nuts and seeds (almonds, cashews, walnuts, pumpkin seeds, flaxseeds, sunflower seeds and chia seeds)

Sugars

100% pure maple syrup or raw honey

Equipment

Flaxseed grinder (either a manual grinder like a pepper mill, or an electric one that is usually sold as a coffee grinder)

Blender

Food processor

1 standard measuring cup. If you don't have a measuring cup try to use a standard mug. Just make sure you use the same one each time!

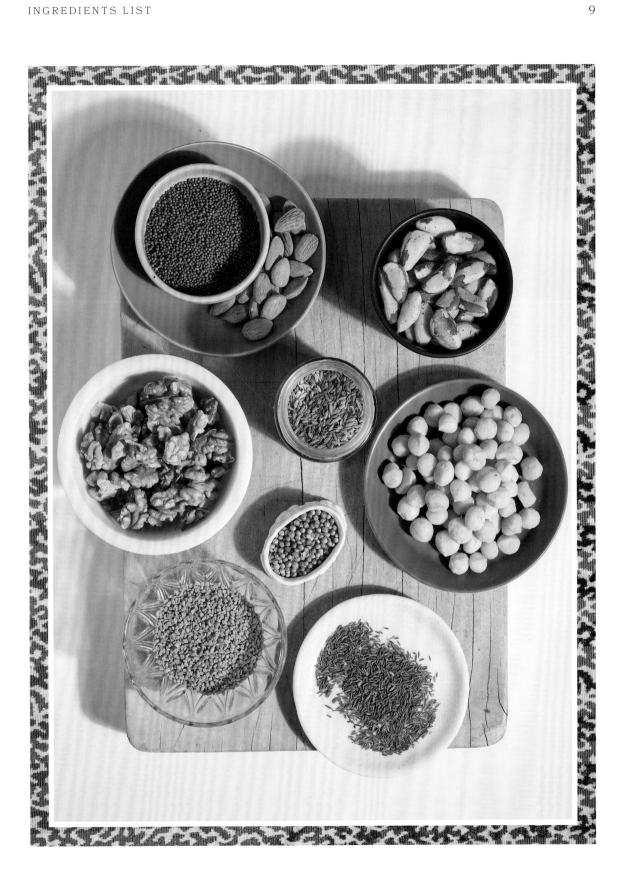

2-Week Plan

Week 1

	Monday	Tuesday	Wednesday
Breakfast	Super-speedy breakfast	Muesli	Cottage cheese toast with avocado
Lunch	Pasta with beans	One-tray salad	Pasta with beans
Dinner	Spiced chickpea coconut curry	Soba noodles with crispy kale	Fish pie with sweet potato mash
Snack	Avocado on rye bread or oat cakes	1 or 2 boiled eggs	Hummus with your choice of crudités
Lifestyle tip	Take at least a 15-minute walk in nature	Leave your phone in a different room to the one where you sleep	Take a 500g (1lb 2oz) Epsom salt bath at least 1 hour before bed

Week 2

	Monday	Tuesday	Wednesday
Breakfast	Super-speedy breakfast	Muesli	Sun-dried tomato butterbeans on toast
Lunch	15-minute pea, mint and butter bean soup	Swedish dill salad	15-minute pea, mint and butter bean soup
Dinner	Vegetable tagine with almond and chickpea quinoa	Miso, ginger, carrot and brown rice stir-fry	Vegetable tagine with almond and chickpea quinoa
Snack	Baba ghanoush with your choice of crudités	1 or 2 boiled eggs	Dark chocolate bark
Lifestyle tip	Take four deep breaths (in through the nose, out through the mouth) before eating	Drink 2 litres of water	No social media between 9pm and 9am

Thursday	Friday	Saturday	Sunday
Super-speedy breakfast	Muesli	Loaded breakfast hash	Spinach banana pancakes
One-tray salad	Pasta with beans	Miso mushroom, avocado and spinach sandwich	Chicken and cauliflower peanut sesame traybake
Spiced chickpea coconut curry	Fish pie with sweet potato mash	Cajun cod with black bean salsa	Walnut meat tacos
Apple with nut butter	Palm-sized serving of nuts	Hummus with your choice of crudités	Dark chocolate bark
Hit your daily steps target	Turn notifications off on all apps in your phone	Read a chapter of a book	Light a scented candle for at least 30 mins to signify 'you' time
Super-speedy breakfast	Muesli	Mushroom shakshuka	Loaded breakfast hash
Swedish dill salad	15-minute pea, mint and butter bean soup	Avocado vegetable panini	Tomato and ricotta tart
Roasted aubergine and tomato pasta	Soy and chilli salmon traybake	Veggie pad Thai noodles	Soy and chilli salmon traybake
Palm-sized serving of nuts	Dark chocolate spread with peanut butter on an oatcake	Baba ghanoush with your choice of crudités	Chocolate and peanut date bites
Not pressing snooze on the alarm, but getting straight up	Do 10 minutes of a meditation app	Hit your daily steps target	Do at least 20 minutes of yoga

1

Focus
on whole
foods

The nutrition industry is full of conflicting advice, but the one principle everyone agrees on is that eating whole foods is good for you. Countless studies show they are great for our gut, they protect our heart and brain, plus they help us to maintain a healthy weight. There is also evidence they can support our mental health.

What are whole foods?

Whole foods, also known as unprocessed or minimally processed foods, are plant-based foods that have undergone minimal processing before eating and are as near to their original state as possible. Some foods, such as fruits and vegetables, are entirely unprocessed, though others, such as ground flours and fermented milk products like yogurt, can also be classified as whole foods.

Whole foods retain more of their natural goodness, in terms of vitamins and fibre, than processed and ultra-processed foods and are generally richer in high-quality complex carbohydrates, meaning they provide slow-release energy. They also contain fewer empty calories from added sugars and trans fats, so you get more nutritional bang for your buck. Examples include:

— **Wholegrains** such as oats, quinoa, buckwheat, corn, rice (black, brown and wild)
— **Nuts** such as almonds, walnuts, pecans, hazelnuts, cashews, peanuts and Brazil nuts
— **Seeds** such as sunflower seeds, chia seeds and pumpkin seeds
— **Pulses and beans** such as lentils, chickpeas, kidney beans, black beans and butter beans
— **Fruits and vegetables** from blueberries to sweet potatoes, and yellow, green and red peppers

Degrees of processing

The NOVA classification system splits all food into four categories, based on how processed they are. The classifications are:

— Unprocessed and minimally processed foods
— Processed culinary ingredients
— Processed food
— Ultra-processed food

Unprocessed and minimally processed foods (group 1)
Unprocessed foods are foods that are in their natural state. Minimally processed foods are natural foods that have been altered by methods that include removal of inedible or unwanted parts, and also processes that include grinding, crushing, filtering, boiling, drying, powdering, fractioning, roasting, non-alcoholic fermentation, pasteurization, chilling, freezing, placing in containers, and vacuum packaging.

Processed culinary ingredients (group 2)
Processed culinary ingredients are calorie-dense foods you rarely eat by themselves, such as oils, butter, sugar and non-caloric ingredients like salt. These ingredients are usually derived from group 1 foods or from foods in their natural state by processes such as pressing, refining and grinding. Some of the methods used to make processed culinary ingredients are mechanical, but the majority are made through industrial processes using chemicals and additives. As a result, some oils in this category are best avoided entirely.

Processed foods (group 3)
Processed foods are typically foods from group 1 to which group 2 foods have been added. They include foods that have been canned or bottled in brine, syrup or oil. They also include some meats like hams and bacon, as well as smoked products, fresh breads and cheeses to which salt has been added. The easiest way to tell the difference between group 1 foods and group 3 foods is to scan the label to see if any group 2 foods have been added.

Processed foods can become a cause for concern when excessive oil, sugar or salt are added and/or they are overconsumed. When consumed in moderation, and in the case of processed meats only occasionally, they can form part of a healthy balanced diet.

Ultra-processed foods (group 4)
Ultra-processed foods are created by a series of industrial techniques and processes consisting of formulations of ingredients, usually involving industrially produced chemicals and additives.

Label reading

If a food doesn't come in a packet, the chances are it isn't processed. If it does, turn the packet over and read the label. Generally, the more ingredients on the back of the packet, the more has been done to it. Watch out for marketing buzzwords and ask yourself how far from its original state is this item.

Sugar

The WHO recommends that adults and children reduce their daily intake of free sugars to less than 10 per cent of their total energy intake. And suggests a further reduction to below 5 per cent or roughly 25 grams (6 teaspoons) per day would provide additional health benefits. UK health guidelines state a daily intake of no more than 30g (1oz) of free sugars per day.

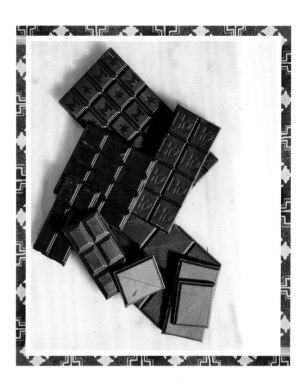

Understanding the distinctions in sugar terminology can help when trying to work out how much sugar is advisable to be consuming per day.

Natural, added, 'free' and total sugars

Natural sugars are the sugars found in fruits, vegetables, dairy and honey. When they are within the cellular structure of foods, such as whole fruit (fructose) and plain milk and yogurt (lactose) they come packaged with vitamins, minerals and, in the case of fruit, fibre and antioxidants.

Added sugar includes all added sugar in whatever form, including table sugar, honey, syrups and nectars that are added to products during manufacture and by the consumer during cooking or at the table.

'Free sugars', according to the WHO refers to monosaccharides (such as glucose or fructose) and disaccharides (such as sucrose or table sugar) added to foods and drinks by the manufacturer, cook or consumer, and sugars naturally present in honey, syrups, fruit juices and fruit juice concentrates. The sugars naturally present in milk and milk products (lactose) and the sugars in the cellular structure of foods are excluded.

Total sugars is the total amount of sugars, and includes naturally occurring and free sugars.

Working out the sugar content of a food is not always straightforward. In the UK, the total sugar content of all manufactured foods is shown on the label as the number of grams of sugar per 100g of the product, with all added sugars declared in the ingredients list on the food label. The US has started to introduce 'added sugars' on the labels of pre-packaged food and drink products, and the US Food & Drug Administration (FDA) is continuing to work with manufacturers to meet these new labelling requirements. 'Added sugars' are calculated based on product manufacturers' proprietary recipes as a baseline.

Marketing buzzwords

Sugar free
In the UK and Europe, this means the food must contain less than 0.5g of sugar per 100g (3½oz). In the US, according to the FDA, 'sugar free' means the item must contain less than 0.5g of sugar per Reference Amounts Customarily Consumed (RACC) and per labelled serving.

No added sugar
In the UK and Europe, when manufacturers claim a food has 'no added sugars,' it can contain naturally occurring sugar but cannot be processed with any sugar or any other food used for its sweetening properties. If sugars are naturally present in the food, the following indication should also appear on the label: 'contains naturally occurring sugars'. In the US, according to the FDA, products with the 'no added sugar' claim can also contain naturally occurring sugars and cannot be processed with any sugar or sugar-containing ingredients, although they can contain sugar alcohol or artificial sweeteners.

Low/Light(er)
This means that this product contains 30 per cent less sugar or fat than a comparable one. Often fat has been removed and replaced with sugar and other unwanted additives, so these are not necessarily a healthier option.

High protein/fibre
For a product to claim to be 'high in protein', at least 20 per cent of the calories must come from protein. To be a 'source of protein', 12 per cent of the calories must be from protein. To be high in fibre there must be 6g (⅛oz) of fibre per 100g (3½oz) – with adults recommended to consume 30g/1oz fibre per day.

Traditional/Farmhouse
Not to be confused with organic. Quite often images of farms, nature and home cooking are used when really the products are highly processed, contain additives and are mass-produced on an industrial scale.

Whole vs Processed

Eat	Fruit and vegetables	Meat/fish/eggs (consume moderately)	Dairy (consume moderately)
	Fresh and frozen fruits	Grass-fed lean meats	Hard cheese and cottage cheese
	Fresh and frozen vegetables	chicken fingers	Plain yogurt
	Unsalted nuts	Fresh fish/shellfish	Full-fat or semi-skimmed milk
		Eggs	
Avoid	Fruit and vegetable juices	Bacon, sausages, hot dogs, deli meats	Highly processed cheeses, such as cheese strings
	Fruits canned in syrup	Fish sticks	Sweetened or flavoured yogurts
	Fruit snacks such as fruit leathers/roll ups		Ice cream
	Vegetable and potato crisps/chips		
	Salted/seasoned nuts		

FACT CHECK

'Healthy sugars' – Refined sugars vs refined sugar-free

There are now a ton of sugary alternatives on the market, labelled as 'refined sugar-free', advertising themselves as a 'healthy' alternative to white table sugar. More specifically, honey, agave syrup, date syrup and coconut sugar etc. However, 'refined sugar free' is not a synonym for 'healthy'. So, whether a sugar is refined or 'refined sugar free' doesn't matter, if it is a free sugar it still contributes towards your daily sugar allowance.

More information on sugar on page 53.

It's about adding more to your diet, not taking away

It's much easier to tell someone to stop eating something than to start including things, so the diet industry has always been very focused on what people can take out of their diets. However, a restrictive diet is never going to be sustainable in the long term as our body needs a diverse range of nutrients to function optimally. It's also a lot more fun to add in rather than take away. So, start adding in more wholegrains, vegetables, seeds and nuts!

Focusing on eating more of what's good for you will also mean there is less space for junk foods and refined products. That doesn't mean you can't still enjoy cakes and chocolate but by increasing your awareness of what you're eating and changing the balance towards whole foods you'll find that processed and ultra-processed junk foods no longer make up as large a part of your diet.

Calorie counting

Digesting and absorbing food uses about 10 per cent of our daily energy expenditure, but this percentage changes with the type of food you eat. Protein uses the most energy with 20–30 per cent of calories lost in digestion. High-fibre foods such as carbohydrates represent more calories than are used largely because fibre can pass undigested through the body. On average, 5–10 per cent of calories are lost in digestion. Fat loses the least calories, with about 5–10 per cent lost through digestion and absorption. We need some fat in our diet to help us absorb fat-soluble vitamins A, D, E and K. Fats are also a source of essential fatty acids, which the body cannot make itself and are crucial for it to function optimally.

It's worth noting that processed foods take less energy to digest and absorb compared with whole foods. So 100 calories of processed food, such as crumpets, biscuits or cake, have a larger calorific impact on the body than 100 calories of a whole food, as fewer calories are used digesting and absorbing them. Consequently, 100 calories of processed food is more net calories than 100 calories of whole food (plus it is usually missing important nutrients).

How many calories we extract from our food can also depend on:
— How we prepare food
— Which bacteria are in our gut
— What species/type of food we eat
— Individual metabolism

All of which means that I am not a fan of calorie counting. It has a place in some situations, but in most cases if the focus is placed on improving the overall quality of your diet, then the desired health benefits will follow without the need for it. Additionally, just because a food is low-calorie does not mean that it is better for you. Quite often, calories are lost at the expense of nutrients, so these low-calorie foods have little nutritional value.

The importance of fibre

Fibre is a type of carbohydrate that is not broken down in the small intestine but instead passes through to the large intestine where it acts as 'food' for the good bacteria in our gut. When breaking down fibre, these good bacteria produce a range of beneficial compounds called short chain fatty acids (SCFAs).

SCFAs perform the following functions:
— Provide fuel for our gut lining
— Contribute to blood sugar balance. It's important
   to keep blood sugar levels within your target range
   throughout the day to help prevent or delay serious
   long-term health problems, such as heart disease,
   vision loss and kidney disease. Staying within your
   target range can also help improve your energy and
   mood. Target blood sugar levels differ for everyone,
   but generally speaking: if you monitor yourself at
   home with a self-testing kit – a normal target is
   4–7mmol/l before eating and under 8.5–9mmol/l
   2 hours after a meal.
— Help food to move through the large intestine.
— Support immunity, stimulate the release of gut
   hormones and directly impact fat tissue.

In addition, fibre also:
— Slows the emptying of our stomach, which makes
   us feel fuller for longer and helps prevent blood
   sugar spikes.
— Contributes to bulking out our stool, making it
   easier to pass.
— Thickens the contents of our gut, which gives our
   gut lining more to work with and helps to regulate
   when we need to go to the loo.
— Binds to other compounds, which can help prevent
   blood sugar spikes and reduce cholesterol levels.

Fibre is your gut microbiome's favourite food and a
happy, well-fed gut microbiome will benefit just about
every organ in your body, including your heart, mental
and skin health.

How much fibre do you need?

Most of us are getting less than 20g (⅔oz) a day.
Guidelines recommend 30g (1oz), but really the
more the better! Make sure, though, you increase
fibre steadily, and that you stay well hydrated, or you
could experience symptoms such as bloating and
constipation.

Where do we get fibre?

Fibre is the backbone of whole foods. Each plant-based
food group (wholegrains, nuts, seeds, pulses and beans,
fruit and veg) contains different types of fibre. The

evidence shows that the more diverse the range of fibre
we consume, the more diverse our gut microbiome,
and a diverse microbiome is associated with the best
health outcomes. So, getting as many different types of
fibre into your diet as possible is key to good gut health.

A good way of ensuring you maximise your fibre intake
is to eat the skin of fruit and vegetables as it contains
a lot of the nutrients, especially fibre and antioxidants.

TERMINOLOGY

What is an antioxidant?

Antioxidants are molecules that neutralize
free radicals, which are unstable molecules that
can harm your cells and can contribute to the
development of many chronic health problems,
such as cardiovascular and inflammatory diseases
and cancer.

7 ways to boost your fibre

1. Add flavour and texture to salads by popping in
    beans or pulses.

2. Sprinkle mixed seeds on cereal, eggs and toast.

3. Don't peel your fruit or veg.

4. Stir beans or pulses into soups.

5. Switch from white to brown/wholegrain bread.

6. Snack on nuts or seeds.

7. If cooking with mince, substitute half for
    beans or lentils.

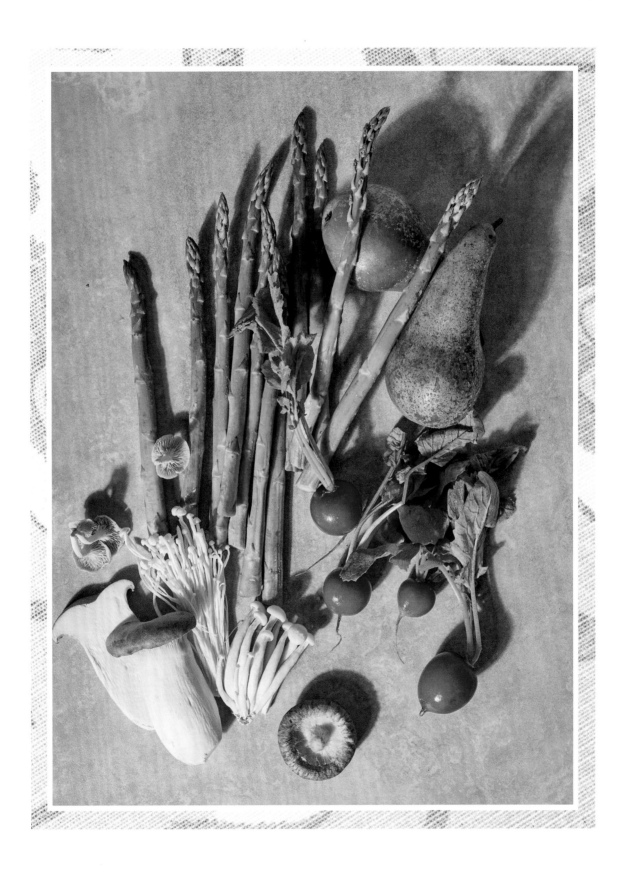

Ways to improve how you food shop

Fruit and veg

A nutritionist advising people to eat more fruit and veg is a bit of a cliché, but they really are the best. Not only are they packed full of fibre, vitamins and minerals, but they also contain health-boosting chemical compounds called phytonutrients, of which there are thousands of different types.

The more varieties and forms of fruits and veg you can get into your diet the better. Different colours of fruits and veg denote a different array of nutrients, and we want as broad a spectrum as possible to make sure our bodies are functioning optimally. Different forms are all great – including canned, fresh and frozen. Buy whatever is easiest but try mixing it up! Five a day is great but really, we want to be aiming for between 7–10 a day.

Wholegrains

Wholegrains include oats, quinoa, buckwheat, corn, rice (black, brown and wild), spelt, barley and bulgur wheat. When used to make bread, pasta and noodles, they are more nutrient-dense than white versions but are not quite as good as when they are in their original, unrefined form.

Unrefined wholegrains are associated with several health benefits as they contain more fibre and nutrients than their refined counterparts. They take longer to digest and be absorbed so help to support good blood sugar balance. Their additional fibre content means you are also likely to find them more filling, so you may find you eat less as a result. The Western diet often bases meals around starchy carbs, but it's important to make sure that these don't take the place of fruit and veg on your plate.

Meat

Historically, meat was a treat, but it has become an everyday food. Research suggests that a healthy diet should include low to moderate amounts of poultry and little to no red or processed meat. Cured meats are particularly concerning. Ham, bacon and salami contain nitrate-based preservatives and high amounts of salt, both of which are associated with poor health outcomes, such as an increased risk of some cancers and heart disease. White meat, such as chicken, is often seen as a healthy alternative, but even this should only be eaten sparingly.

If you plan well, it is perfectly possible to have a nutritious meat-free diet, but if you choose to eat meat, opt for well-raised animals and consume it in moderate amounts. One way of reducing your consumption is to aim for more meat-free days per week than those with meat, and to eat red or processed meats as only a very occasional treat. I would also recommend choosing organic meat, if possible. Although it is more expensive, that cost is reflected in the quality of the meat, which tends to have a higher nutritional content. For example, organic livestock-rearing often correlates with higher levels of omega-3 fatty acids. The additional cost can also act as an incentive to reduce your consumption.

On your meat-free days, try to stay away from meat replacement products – such as Quorn, vegan bacon and sausages etc – as they are often highly processed. Instead, aim to use whole foods, such as beans and pulses or, occasionally, tofu (which is not a whole food).

FACT CHECK

What is the difference between the words 'grass-fed' and 'pasture-fed'?

In the UK, the words 'grass-fed' can be used to describe food from animals that have spent only part of their time out grazing in the fields or eating conserved grass. The rest of the time they will have been fed other less natural feeds, such as cereals or the by-products of human food manufacturing like bread and biscuit waste. If you want to make sure the meat products you are buying have come from animals raised purely on pasture, look for the 'Pasture for Life' logo. This food is guaranteed to have been produced to the highest welfare standards and is truly pasture-fed.

Fish

Fish is a great source of healthy protein and nutrients, particularly oily fish, such as sardines, mackerel, anchovies, salmon and herring, which are rich in omega-3s. Research on the health benefits of omega-3 polyunsaturated fatty acids EPA and DHA is wide ranging and well established. For example, evidence shows that oily fish eaters have more grey matter in their brains, which is the tissue most linked to memory.

People whose diets include regular fish consumption are generally associated with a lower risk of becoming overweight and obese. Oily fish is the best way to ensure good omega-3 intake; the UK and Europe health guidelines recommend eating at least two portions of fish a week, with at least one being oily (but no more if you are pregnant). The Dietary Guidelines for Americans recommends at least 226g (8 ounces) of fish per week (based on a 2,000 calorie diet) and less for children. Those who might become or are pregnant or breastfeeding should eat between 226–340g (8–12 ounces) of a variety of fish per week, from choices that are lower in mercury. If you don't eat a lot of oily fish, you may want to consider taking a high-quality omega-3 supplement (always look for a high EPA and DHA content) and increasing your consumption of plant sources of omega-3s, such as flaxseeds, chia seeds and walnuts. However, research shows that plant sources of omega-3s aren't as well converted as fish sources.

When buying fish, choose sustainably-caught wild fish, or organic farmed fish. Unprocessed frozen and canned fish can be just as nutritious as fresh but take note of what the fish has been canned with and ideally choose one that has been canned in water or extra virgin olive oil, as brine contains a lot of salt and other fats are not as healthy. Smaller fish, such as sardines and mackerel, are preferable to big ones, such as tuna. This is because larger fish tend to be further up the food chain and will have eaten smaller fish. As a result, they often have higher levels of heavy metals and other toxins, having ingested their own as well as those of the fish they have eaten.

Eggs

I love eggs! They are high in protein and other important vitamins and minerals, including vitamins B2, B5, B12 and D and choline. It's true they contain high levels of dietary cholesterol, but multiple studies have shown they have a minimal impact on blood cholesterol levels, especially when consumed as part of a healthy diet. Always opt for organic or free-range eggs as they will be of a higher quality and more nutritious, plus it is much better for the welfare of the birds. Organic or free-range options offer a more natural and stimulating existence to egg-laying birds. The eggs from grass-fed birds also have higher levels of vitamin E and offer about double the amounts omega-3 fats.

Legumes and pulses

A diet rich in legumes and pulses has been shown to be associated with better health outcomes, such as a lower risk of cancer, obesity and cardiovascular disease, as well a long and healthy life. There is a fascinating body of work that highlights the concept of 'Blue Zone' regions of the world in which people have low rates of chronic disease and live longer than anywhere else. Researchers identified several factors that Blue Zones have in common, one of which is a diet that is 95 per cent plant-based and includes legumes and pulses daily.

Legumes and pulses are a good source of protein and fibre, which means they are going to fill you up, and are low in saturated fat. Legumes and pulses may cause bloating if they are not properly cooked. Dried versions, which have been soaked and then cooked often tend to be digested more easily than canned, as many brands cook them in the can, which isn't as good. Dried lack the convenience of canned, though, so experiment with a few brands to find one that suits you.

Dairy

Unless you are lactose-intolerant, minimally processed dairy products should be included as part of a healthy diet as dairy, although not essential, offers valuable nutrients, such as protein and calcium. Personally, I have one serving of natural yogurt most days, but only very occasionally consume cheese or have milk in my tea. I also use extra virgin olive oil rather than butter, but these are just my preferences!

Nuts and seeds

Although small, nuts and seeds are amazing nutrition powerhouses that you can add to almost every dish. Sorely underutilized in the Western diet, they are fantastic sources of protein, healthy fats and key vitamins and minerals such as selenium (Brazil nuts), omega 3s (walnuts) and magnesium (almonds).

Portion sizes for adults

Thumb sized

Index finger

Fist-sized

Palm-sized

Fruit and veg
1 portion

1 fist-sized serving

1 large handful of spinach

1 medium tomato

1 medium apple

Protein
1 portion

1 palm-sized serving

half a handful of fish / 140g (5oz)

120g (4¼oz) cooked beans/lentils

1 palm-sized serving nuts and/or seeds

80g (2¾oz) tofu

Carbohydrates
1 portion

1 fist-sized serving

1 fist-sized baked potato or sweet potato

2 medium slices of bread

2 handfuls of dried rice/pasta/quinoa

Dairy and dairy alternatives
1 portion

200ml (7fl oz) semi-skimmed milk

3 tablespoons natural yogurt

1 index finger-length of cheese / 30g (1oz)

Fat
1 portion

1 dessertspoon/10ml (¼ teaspoon) oil drizzled on salads or to cook a meal

Healthy swaps

Instead of white pasta	Brown pasta, brown rice pasta, chickpea pasta or green pea pasta
Instead of white bread	Brown/wholegrain bread, rye bread, brown sourdough
Instead of couscous	Quinoa, buckwheat
Instead of white rice	Brown rice, wild rice
Instead of crisps or a cereal bar	Raw unsalted nuts, seeds, raisins, dried apricots
Instead of a sugary breakfast cereal	Whole rolled oats

Action points

1. **Plan ahead**
Choose three (or more!) healthy recipes/meals for the week ahead that share similar whole foods.

Write a list before you go shopping and stick to it. Try not to be tempted by flashy signs and offers when you're in the supermarket!

Don't shop when you're hungry.

2. **Buy whole**
Be clear in your mind about what whole foods are. Ask yourself, is this food made by man or nature?

If in doubt, remember to read the label. The simpler and fewer the number of ingredients, the less likely the item is to be processed.

3. **Make animal products a treat**
Include animal products in your diet if you would like to but be aware that the more you eat, the less room you will have for fibre-rich plant foods.

Aim for more days without them than with them.

Keep red meat consumption low, ideally to a maximum of one palm-sized portion a week.

4. **Add legumes and pulses**
Try them in salads, soups and curries.

Experiment with chickpea pasta, or green pea pasta.

5. **Aim for at least half of your plate to be veg and fruits,** a quarter protein foods and a quarter wholegrain foods

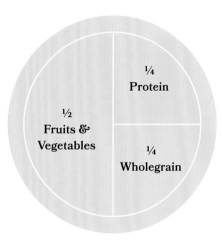

¼
Protein

½
Fruits &
Vegetables

¼
Wholegrain

6. **Make healthy swaps**
Increase your fibre and nutrient intake by choosing whole foods over processed. For example, swap white for brown, sugary yogurt for natural, make your pasta sauce rather than buying it.

Be
Diverse

A varied diet is the key both to good gut health and to good overall health as the bacteria in our gut need a diverse range of fibres to feed off, and our body needs a diverse range of nutrients to function. Having reduced bacterial diversity in your gut means that you are more susceptible to disease, whereas with a diverse microbiota, you are more likely to bounce back from unhealthy fluctuations in your diet and to be able to withstand the environmental and biological challenges of daily life. Time and again I see people in my clinic who eat only from a restricted repertoire of foods, unaware of how they could be limiting their health.

The number of different plant species we eat has a significant impact on the bacterial diversity of our gut. However, modern food retailing and farming practices mean that the fruit and veg we eat today is much more limited in terms of diversity and variety than that eaten by our forebears. Modern processing and the need for global food availability has removed the natural variety from our diet. For example, a standardized variety of orange carrot is grown at the expense of other varieties. The consequence of decisions like this, according to the United Nations, is that 75 per cent of plant diversity has been lost since 1900. All of which means that we need to work hard to put that variety back in.

Eat a rainbow – 5 a day (ideally 7–10 a day)

The body needs a broad spectrum of nutrients to ensure it has everything it needs to function optimally. Different colours of fruits and vegetables contain a different array of nutrients, so eating a rainbow of foods daily provides the variety of vitamins, minerals, antioxidants and phytochemicals needed for healthy skin, muscles and cells, as well as to fight infection and to help support a balanced immune system and a diverse and healthy gut microbiome.

Although the recommended amount of fruit and veg you should eat is five portions a day, in reality it should be 7–10 a day, so aim for at least one serving from each of the columns below every day. (See page 22 for portion sizes.)

Green		Purple/ Blue		Brown/ White
Artichoke	Spring greens	Aubergine	Peaches	
Asparagus	Watercress	Beetroot	Pineapple	
Bok choy		Blackberries	Pumpkin	
Broccoli	**Red**	Blueberries	Squash	
Brussels sprouts	Cherries	Plums	Sweet potato	
Cabbage	Radicchio	Purple asparagus		
Celery	Radishes	Purple grapes	**Brown/ White**	
Collard greens	Raspberries	Red cabbage	Bananas	
Courgette	Red apples		Brown pears	
Cucumber	Red chillies		Cauliflower	
Green pepper	Red grapes	**Orange/Yellow**	Dates	
Kale	Red onion	Carrots	Garlic	
Kiwi	Red pepper	Apricots	Ginger	
Leeks	Rhubarb	Cantaloupe melon	Mushrooms	
Lettuce	Strawberries	Corn	Onions	
Okra	Tomato	Grapefruit	Parsnips	
Pak choi	Watermelon	Lemons	Potatoes	
Rocket		Mangoes	Turnip	
Spinach		Nectarines	White peaches	
		Oranges		

10 ways to diversify your diet

1. **Experiment with different wholegrains.** For example, use quinoa instead of rice, oats instead of store-bought cereal, or try adding spelt or barley into soups or salads. If you can't find anywhere that stocks more unusual wholegrains, order them online.
2. **Try different preparation methods.** If you roasted your vegetables yesterday, try steaming them today, and eating them raw tomorrow.
3. **Make sure you have every colour in your shopping trolley,** and at least three colours on your plate. (See the Eat a Rainbow table for guidance, on the opposite page.)
4. **Leave a jar of mixed seeds on your kitchen or dining table** to remind you to add them to your food.
5. **Buy pre-mixed combinations** of fruits, veg, nuts, seeds or pulses and legumes.
6. **Keep a range of dried herbs on your kitchen counter** to remind you to use them. And try adding them to your dishes. Opt for mixed herbs to start with, then add more to your collection as you go along. For example, cinnamon on porridge or mixed herbs in a salad dressing.
7. **Choose one day of the week to be 'try a new plant-food day'.**
8. **Roast a big batch of mixed veg** (for example, red onions, peppers and squash) at the beginning of the week and keep in the fridge or freezer. That way you will always have something on hand.
9. **Try one new recipe a week.**
10. **Eat seasonally.** Try adding a seasonal ingredient to your shopping list or booking a regular delivery with a veg box scheme. Eating seasonally brings a natural diversity to your diet, taking you on a journey around different plant foods. You'll also be eating fruits and vegetables when they are at their most nutritious (and most local). If you ever don't know what to do with a vegetable, try adding it to a soup or pasta.

Up your polyphenols

Polyphenols (aka phytochemicals) are chemicals found in plants that protect them against bacteria, viruses and fungi. The action of phytochemicals varies according to the colour and type of food. They may act as antioxidants, nutrient protectors or prevent carcinogens (cancer-causing agents) from forming. An antioxidant helps defend your cells from damage caused by potentially harmful molecules known as free radicals. When free radicals accumulate, they may cause a state known as oxidative stress, which can damage your DNA and other important structures in your cells, drive inflammation, accelerate the ageing process and contribute to a number of health conditions.

Foods high in polyphenols

Fruit
Blueberries, blackcurrants, plums, cherries, blackberries, strawberries, raspberries, prunes, black grapes, apples

Vegetables and legumes
Asparagus, broccoli, spinach, red onion, chicory, artichokes, green olives, black olives, white beans, black beans

Nuts and seeds
Flaxseeds, hazelnuts, pecans, almonds, chestnuts

Herbs and spices
Caraway, cinnamon, ginger, rosemary, capers, celery seeds, cloves, sages, oregano, thyme, basil, peppermint, rosemary, spearmint, star anise, ginger, curry powder

Fats
Extra virgin olive oil

Drinks
Filtered coffee, black tea, green tea, cocoa (at least 75 per cent cocoa), red wine

30 plant points

While 5 a day (but ideally 7–10 a day) is a great place to start, it ignores the different types of plant foods our gut bacteria microbiota needs to flourish. In an international gut microbiome project, researchers found that eating 30 or more different types of plants a week supports the gut's bacterial diversity and barrier strength, by providing a diverse range of vitamins, minerals and phytonutrients, and is also linked to the production of short chain fatty acids (SCFAs), which are associated with numerous health benefits (see page 18).

Food diversity assessment

What counts?
All vegetables, fruits, wholegrains, pulses and legumes, nuts and seeds are 1 point per portion, with herbs and spices ¼ point per portion.

Over the course of one week, note down the different types of plants you eat and calculate the total at the end.

This list is not exhaustive, so if there are other plants you have eaten that are not mentioned, add them in the other box for that section.

1   2   3   4   5   6   7

Veg (fresh or frozen)

○○○○○○○ **Cruciferous vegetables** (brassica family): rocket, broccoli, broccoli sprouts, Brussels sprouts, cabbage, cauliflower, collard greens, kale, pak choi, bok choy, swede, radish, turnip, watercress

○○○○○○○ **Leafy greens:** spinach, lettuce, spring greens

○○○○○○○ **Salad:** radishes, celery, cucumber, radicchio

○○○○○○○ **Alliums:** spring onions, onions, leeks, garlic

○○○○○○○ **Root veg:** carrots, beetroot, parsnips, celeriac, radishes, beetroot, turnip but not potatoes

○○○○○○○ Bell peppers, red chilli

○○○○○○○ Peas

○○○○○○○ Mushrooms

○○○○○○○ Tomatoes

○○○○○○○ Avocado

○○○○○○○ Aubergines, courgettes

1   2   3   4   5   6   7

○○○○○○○ Corn, sweetcorn

○○○○○○○ Asparagus, artichoke, celery

○○○○○○○ Other

Fruit (fresh or frozen)

○○○○○○○ **Citrus fruit:** lemons, oranges, grapefruit

○○○○○○○ **Berries:** blueberries, strawberries, raspberries, blackberries

○○○○○○○ **Tree fruit:** apples, pears, plums, peaches, nectarines, apricots, cherries, grapes

○○○○○○○ Bananas

○○○○○○○ Kiwi, mangoes, pineapple

○○○○○○○ Melon, watermelon

○○○○○○○ Other

1 2 3 4 5 6 7   1 2 3 4 5 6 7

Wholegrains

○○○○○○○ 100 per cent rolled oats

○○○○○○○ Rice (black, brown or wild
are generally more nutritious
then white)

○○○○○○○ Oatcakes

○○○○○○○ Quinoa, buckwheat, spelt,
barley, bulgur wheat

○○○○○○○ Wholewheat flour

○○○○○○○ Wholegrain/brown rice pasta

○○○○○○○ Other

Pulses and legumes
(canned or cooked
from dried)

○○○○○○○ Chickpeas

○○○○○○○ Lentils

○○○○○○○ Beans (black, butter,
cannellini, kidney, pinto,
chickpeas, edamame, mung)

○○○○○○○ Other

Nuts and seeds
(not processed, unsalted)

○○○○○○○ Almonds, walnuts, pecans,
hazelnuts, cashews, peanuts,
brazil nuts

○○○○○○○ Other

Herbs and spices
(dried or fresh)

○○○○○○○ Cinnamon, cloves, nutmeg,
star anise, ginger

○○○○○○○ Paprika, chilli powder/flakes,
curry powder, cumin

○○○○○○○ Parsley, coriander, basil,
oregano, sage, rosemary

○○○○○○○ Peppermint

○○○○○○○ Other

< 10   **Try to get diversifying**
10–19   **Add more diversity to your diet**
20–29   **Keep going!**
30+   **You are one diverse person**

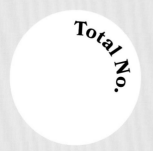

Total No.

Fruits   Vegetables   Wholegrains

Pulses   Nuts   Herbs
and legumes   and seeds   and spices

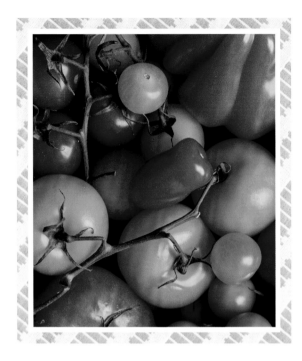

Your cooking method matters

How you prepare food can significantly alter its nutritional content. Although cooking improves the digestion and absorption of nutrients, it may reduce levels of some vitamins and minerals. So, it's good to vary your preparation methods.

Raw
It's great to include raw foods in your diet as most vitamins and minerals are in their most available form in this state. However, some nutrients, like the antioxidant beta carotene in carrots, are increased with cooking. So, it's good to vary what state you eat things in.

Microwaving
Preserves most nutrients due to short cooking times.

Steaming
Does not require any fat and is one of the best cooking methods for preserving nutrients.

Baking
Virtually fat free and a great way to retain nutrients.

Boiling
Vitamin C and B vitamins are heat-sensitive so some can be reduced during cooking.

Roasting
Most vitamin losses are minimal, apart from B vitamins.

Pan-frying
Has little effect on the mineral content of the food and preserves vitamin C and B vitamins. The high temperature and short transit time of the frying process causes less loss of heat-sensitive vitamins than other types of cooking. Pan-frying is healthier than deep-frying or shallow-frying, as while you're using oil in the pan, you're not submerging the food in oil.

Deep-frying
I wouldn't recommend this cooking method. Fat enters the food and deep-frying can add 2–3 times the calories of boiling or baking.

Waste not, want not

Save yourself some work and forget peeling your fruit and veg. As well as reducing food waste, eating the peel has health benefits, as the skin contains many of the nutrients, especially fibre and antioxidants. Think skin on when roasting a butternut squash or (sweet) potatoes, pop celery leaves in a salad, scrub rather than peel those carrots, don't throw away your broccoli stalks and eat the leaves of the cauliflower as well.

Avoid/restrict items that limit gut diversity

Ultra-processed foods
These include crisps, sweets, baked goods and ready meals. They are responsible for many of the unwanted calories in our diets. They have been stripped of much of the original food's fibre (and we know how important fibre is for us gut health from page 18), plus they contain added salt (it's estimated that three-quarters of the salt in our diet comes from processed

and ultra-processed foods), sugar and unwanted fats, chemicals and additives, which can disrupt the gut microbiome.

Salt

Recent evidence suggests that our gut microbiota may play a role in the link between salt and high blood pressure, with several studies finding high salt intake decreases certain health-supporting gut bacteria. The World Health Organization (WHO) recommends that adults restrict salt intake to 5g (⅛oz) per day. UK health guidelines recommend no more than 6g (⅛oz) per day. Watch out for foods such as soy sauce, pickled vegetables, processed meats and processed foods such as snack bars, ready meals, biscuits, cakes, crisps and bread. And check labels, where salt is often listed as sodium. If it is, multiply the sodium content by 2.5 for the salt content. The easiest way to reduce salt intake is to cut down on processed foods and reduce the amount you season your food. You'll find your taste buds adapt fairly quickly and the less you add salt to food, the less you will notice.

Alcohol

The bacteria in our gut help us to metabolize alcohol, which is why we all tolerate it in different ways, having more or less helpful bacteria will impact how effectively you detoxify alcohol. While moderate alcohol consumption may have some positive health impacts, the risks of drinking to excess are well established. Red wine can contain polyphenols, which your gut bugs love, but this is not a reason to drink it, as too much will quickly outweigh any benefits. Excess alcohol can inhibit the production of digestive enzymes and juices, making it more difficult to digest food. Partially digested food can cause excess fermentation in the gut, which often leads to bloating and loose stools. Additionally, excess alcohol can also cause inflammation in the gut as well as result in bacterial overgrowth and dysbiosis.

There is no official World Health Organisation guidance on maximum alcohol intake, so countries have gone their own ways. UK health guidelines are that adults should not regularly drink more than 14 units of alcohol per week, ideally less. UK guidelines are controversially the same for both genders and make it one of the lowest recommended upper limits for alcohol consumption by men in the world. Australian guidelines are also the same for both genders and recommend healthy adults should drink no more than 10 standard drinks a week (equating to roughly 17.5 units per week). For women, UK guidance is roughly in line with US guidance, which recommends a maximum of 1 drink or less per day for women, equating to about 12.3 units a week. Men in the US however are recommended to limit alcohol to 2 drinks or less per day (roughly 24.5 units). Across Europe guidelines vary widely, with Italy and Spain having some of the highest maximums for men and women (35 and 31.5, and 21 and 21.3 units per week respectively), and Germany some of the lowest, recommending men should not have more than the equivalent of two standard drinks per day and women one drink – but everyone should have two alcohol-free days per week (this equates to 21 and 10.5 units per week for men and women respectively).

Drinking limits around the world

Comparison in equivalent UK units (8g of alcohol) and based on weekly upper limits for women and men.

Country	Women	Men
UK	14	14
US	12.3	24.5
France	17.5	26.3
Ireland	13.75	21.3
Australia	17.5	17.5
Germany	10.5	21
Italy	21	31.5
Spain	21.3	35

Artificial sweeteners

There is a small amount of research to suggest that artificial sweeteners aren't good for the gut microbiome and are responsible for an increase in the type of bacteria associated with obesity. Some artificial sweeteners can also upset the digestive system and come with warnings about their laxative effect.

Added sugar comes in many forms (fructose, sucrose, glucose, fruit juice, honey, maple syrup, high fructose corn syrup). UK health guidelines state a daily intake of no more than 30g (1oz) of added sugar (confusingly also referred to as 'free sugar', see page 15). WHO recommends that no more than 5 per cent of daily energy come from free sugars.

Medications (particularly antibiotics)
Taking antibiotics can dramatically change the amount and type of bacteria in the gut as they can cause good bacteria to die off. This results in a metabolic shift, increasing susceptibility to colonization of bad gut bugs, and stimulating development of antibiotic resistance. Often antibiotics can't be avoided, so if you have to take them, here are some ways to support your gut while doing so.

Antibiotic gut health suggestions:

Choose a probiotic with a) saccharomyces boulardii or b) lactobacillus rhamnosus GG with either a dose of a) 5 billion CFU (colony forming units that bacteria are measured in) twice per day or for b) 6 billion CFU twice per day, start taking as soon as you start the antibiotics and continue for a week after you stop the antibiotics.

Take the probiotic supplement at least 2 hours away from antibiotic medication. Ideally 2 hours after breakfast and dinner.

If you have a weak immune system (e.g. during cancer therapy), always discuss with your healthcare provider first.

Drugs and nicotine
The mechanisms as to how drugs and nicotine disturb the gut microbiota are not as yet fully understood, but research points to a link between them and microbiota dysbiosis (imbalance). Given the other negative health impacts associated with them it would also be wise to avoid them for these reasons too.

A sedentary lifestyle
Research suggests that the microbes in people who exercise regularly produce more short chain fatty acids (SCFAs), which help keep your gut lining healthy and regulate your immune system (amongst other things), than in those who lead a more sedentary lifestyle. This doesn't mean going mad in the gym, but the body likes to move, so whether it's going for a walk, or hitting a class, make sure you do some exercise every day.

Stress
Evidence shows that stress hormones can reshape the gut bacteria's composition and also that the gut microbiota can influence stress-related behaviours. So, it's very much a two-way street, with stress influencing the gut and vice versa. Reducing stress is a lot easier said than done but if you can minimize stress it is really going to help your gut health. Activities that relax you, such as going for a walk, breathing exercises, yoga, meditation or listening to a podcast, activate the parasympathetic nervous system (PNS), which controls your rest and digest response (and aids digestion), as opposed to your sympathetic nervous system (SNS), which is your fight or flight response. The two systems are oppositional and cannot be activated at the same time. In modern life we do a lot to stimulate our SNS but not much to support our PNS. If you're struggling with stress it can be helpful to reflect on what you have done to support your PNS, as adding in more parasympathetic supporting activities could help reduce it.

Action points

Good gut health does not need to be time-consuming or costly (no expensive supplements here):

1. **Eat a rainbow everyday**
   Aim for 7–10 different fruits and vegetables a day. Try to pick as many different colours as possible. Refer to the Eat a Rainbow table (page 26) for suggestions.

2. **Aim for 30 plant points a week**
   Simple changes can make a big difference. See 10 ways to diversify your diet, page 27.

3. **Take the plant-based diversity assessment**
   Doing this on a regular basis will help keep you on track (see pages 28–29).

4. **Eat seasonally and locally**
   This is great for achieving a varied diet and for the environment too.

5. **Avoid/restrict items that limit gut diversity**, such as ultra-processed foods, salt, sugars, alcohol, artificial sweeteners, medications (where possible), being sedentary and stress

What !?

the fat

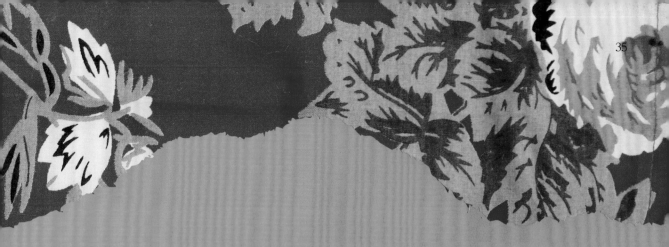

For decades, the diet industry has vilified fat. However, we absolutely need healthy fats in our diet for our bodies to function. Fat helps our body absorb fat-soluble vitamins E, D, A and K, is crucial for cell membrane structure and function, hormone production and brain development and function. The World Health Organization (WHO) tells us that adults need at least 15 per cent of their daily energy from fat – approximately 30g (1oz) a day for women and 40g (1½oz) a day for men.

With awareness growing about the benefits of fats there has also been a rise in conflicting information around what fats we should be consuming. Messaging in the media has often been confusing. Fats are frequently clumped together as one entity when, in fact, there are lots of different types of fat. Additionally, ever since the link between heart disease and fat was established, researchers have spent decades trying to pin down its role in supporting and harming health. Translating the research into simple public messaging is also challenging, and often oversimplified or appearing overwhelming.

Understanding fats

There are two main types of dietary fat: saturated and unsaturated fats. Unsaturated fats are either monounsaturated or polyunsaturated. Most foods contain a mixture of all three.

Saturated fats

These mainly come from animal sources, such as butter, cream, cheese, fatty meats and processed meats, and are the dominant fat in some plant oils, such as coconut oil. They are solid at room temperature, and stable at high temperatures, so therefore less likely to destabilize and damage when they are heated. This damage refers to the molecular structure of the oil being altered and the oil becoming oxidized. This process creates free radicals, which can contribute to the development of many chronic health problems, such as cardiovascular and inflammatory disease and cancer.

Unsaturated fats

Monounsaturated fats (MUFAs)
These are found in oleic acid (which is present in olive oil), avocados, nuts, seeds, rapeseed oil, fish oils and nut oils, and are typically liquid at room temperature. Monounsaturated fats tend to be fairly stable when heated.

Polyunsaturated fats (PUFAs)
These are found in oily fish, walnuts, flaxseeds, sunflower seeds and vegetable oils.

Omega 3 and omega 6 are polyunsaturated fats. The more research there is into omega 3, the more we are coming to understand just how many important roles it has to play in the body and how many health benefits it has. Omega 3 plays a vital role in the immune system, the production of hormones, blood clotting, contraction and relaxation of artery walls and inflammation to name a few.

Artificial trans fats
These are the worst type of fats and, due to concerns they raise LDL cholesterol, are banned in several countries including Denmark, Switzerland, Austria and certain US states, including New York and California. However, a UK ban has not been met with government support, which has preferred to allow food companies to reduce the trans-fat content of their foods on a voluntary basis. Research shows that artificial trans fats raise bad cholesterol, lower good cholesterol and increase the risk of coronary heart disease.

Artificial trans fats are formed through an industrial process that adds hydrogen to vegetable oil, which causes the oil to become solid at room temperature, for example margarine spreads. This partially hydrogenated oil is inexpensive and less likely to spoil, so foods such as pastries and cakes made with it have a longer shelf life. Some restaurants also use partially hydrogenated vegetable oil in their deep-fryers because it doesn't have to be changed as often as other oils do. It is also used as an emulsifier and appears in many other processed foods ,such as hot chocolate mix, ice cream and processed potato products, such as hash browns and crisps.

Some meat and dairy products have a small amount of naturally occurring trans fats. These are not artificial trans fats, and although it's not clear how these trans fats affect health, they are not a cause for concern.

Cholesterol
Cholesterol is a fatty substance that is made in the liver and found in some foods too. Cholesterol plays a vital role in how the body works. There is cholesterol in every cell in your body and it's especially important for your brain, nerves and skin. Evidence shows us that eating eggs or other high cholesterol foods does not elevate blood cholesterol. About 80 per cent of the cholesterol in our bodies is made in the liver, so isn't coming directly from the cholesterol we eat. The body produces cholesterol in much larger quantities then you eat so foods that are high in cholesterol won't affect your blood cholesterol very much.

There are two main types of cholesterol:
LDL cholesterol (Low-density lipoprotein)
This is often called 'bad' cholesterol because too much can lead to health problems. These lipoproteins contain lots of cholesterol. Their job is to deliver cholesterol to the cells where it's needed. But if there's too much LDL cholesterol in your blood it can build up in the arteries, clogging them up.

HDL cholesterol (high-density lipoprotein)

This is often called 'good' cholesterol because it helps prevent disease. It contains lots of protein, and very little cholesterol. HDL cholesterol's job is to carry cholesterol away from the cells, back to the liver, where it can be broken down and removed from the body.

Not the whole cholesterol story

It's not just your total cholesterol that's important and cholesterol test results will include different types of cholesterol. It's possible to have a healthy total cholesterol (TC) number but an unhealthy balance of the different types of cholesterol. If you have a cholesterol test, it is really important that a healthcare professional explains the results to you to prevent unnecessary worry and confusion.

While saturated fat has been shown to raise LDL (bad cholesterol) it also improves the quality of LDL and increases its size, making it less likely to promote heart disease. It also raises the HDL (good cholesterol) and ultimately it is the ratio of total cholesterol to LDL cholesterol, and total cholesterol to LDL particle number and size which are far bigger predictors of heart attacks then LDL itself.

5 tips to improve cholesterol

1. Purple fruits and vegetables are rich in anthocyanins (a group of antioxidants found in red, purple, and blue fruits and vegetables) which may help increase HDL cholesterol levels.
2. Increase consumption of omega-3-rich oily fish, ideally to two times a week. This may help increase HDL cholesterol levels and benefit heart health.
3. Avoid trans fats which can increase total cholesterol and LDL but decrease HDL.
4. Consume pulses and legumes, which have been linked to lower LDL levels.
5. Increase consumption of monounsaturated fats, such as olive oil, avocados and nuts. Monounsaturated fats are healthy because they decrease harmful LDL cholesterol, increase good HDL cholesterol and reduce harmful oxidation.

Type of fat	Sources	Pro	Con	How to use
Saturated	Animal sources such as butter, cream, cheese, fatty meats and processed meats, and are the dominant fat in some plant oils such as coconut oil	Solid at room temperature and stable when heated	Linked to heart disease	Use infrequently as a treat
Unsaturated				
Monounsaturated	Found in oleic acid (which is present in olive oil), avocados, nuts, seeds, rapeseed oil, fish oils and nut oils	Heart healthy	Some of the oils can oxidize easily	Use cold in salad, when cooking at low temperatures and eat as a whole food
Polyunsaturated	Found in oily fish, walnuts, flaxseeds, sunflower seeds, and vegetable oils	Numerous health benefits	Can be unstable when heated	Eat as whole foods
Other				
Artificial trans fats	Largely found in some processed foods and deep-fried foods	None	Linked to heart disease	Never

Where it went wrong

Historically flawed UK government guidelines encouraging us all to move from saturated fats to the 'healthier' unsaturated fats instigated a huge move towards increased consumption of the unsaturated omega 6-rich vegetable oils and trans fat-rich vegetable spreads, which are highly inflammatory to the body and unstable.

Too much omega 6 also counteracts the benefits and availability of anti-inflammatory omega-3 fats. This combination fuels the body's inflammatory pathways and subsequent inflammatory diseases. Omega 6 and omega 3 must be consumed in balance for optimal health.

So is fat bad for us?

The idea that 'fat is bad' has been widely discredited. Fat is crucial for our health. It's important to remember that whole foods do not consist of one type of fat. Nature presents us with saturated, monounsaturated and polyunsaturated all together. For example, olive oil is around 75 per cent monounsaturated fat, 14 per cent saturated fat, and 11 per cent polyunsaturated fat.

While evidence on how much saturated fat we should consume is by no means conclusive, a majority of experts agree that too much saturated fat is bad for our heart, but that doesn't mean avoiding it entirely. The World Health Organization advises intake of saturated fat should be limited to no more than 10 per cent of total energy intake, and intake of trans fats should be less the 1 per cent of total energy intake, with a shift in fat consumption away from saturated fats and trans-fats to unsaturated fats, with a goal of eliminating industrially produced trans-fats entirely.

Organizations such as the British Heart Foundation and the American Heart Association advise replacing saturated fat with unsaturated fat to lower the risk of heart disease. With the focus on including both mono- and polyunsaturated fats in our diet, particularly omega-3 fatty acids (which are associated with numerous health benefits). This is also supported by the UK government's Scientific Advisory Committee on Nutrition, which concluded in 2019 that reducing saturated fat and replacing it with polyunsaturated fats reduces the risk of heart attack and stroke, while replacing saturated fat with monounsaturated fat lowers LDL cholesterol.

Getting good fat in our diet

Essentially, this means increasing omega 3-rich foods and decreasing saturated fat-rich foods. So, avoid artificial trans fats, limit saturated fats to 10–11 per cent and consume moderate amounts of mono- and polyunsaturated fats, particularly omega 3-rich foods, and ideally from whole foods. Be aware, though, that simply increasing omega 3s alone won't overcome a bad diet or one with too much saturated fat.

Some of the best foods for omega-3 fatty acids are oily fish, such as SMASH-T (salmon, mackerel, anchovies, sardines, herring and trout). The best vegetarian sources of omega 3 are omega-3 eggs, chia seeds and flaxseeds (try to buy these seeds whole and grind them yourself as they oxidize quickly once ground).

Some of the foods containing the highest amounts of saturated fats are meat, dairy and vegetable oils. Many people consume an excess of these.

5 ways to avoid artificial trans fats

1. Avoid deep-fried foods. Choose grilled, steamed or baked instead.
2. Avoid takeaways as some restaurants use partially hydrogenated vegetable oil in their deep-fryers.
3. Avoid processed foods, such as breaded or crumb-coated foods.
4. Avoid commercially baked goods, such as cakes and pastries.
5. Eat more wholegrains, pulses and legumes and fruits and vegetables as these contain no artificial trans fats.

5 ways to limit saturated fats

1. Swap butter on your toast for a drizzle of extra virgin olive oil or mashed avocado.
2. Swap butter on your vegetables for extra virgin olive oil and or/lemon juice.
3. Swap cream for blitzed up soaked cashews nuts, almonds or sunflower seeds. You could also use nut butters.
4. Swap cheese for toasted crumbled nuts, roasted seeds, anchovies or olives. Nutritional yeast can be used as a seasoning to add a cheese flavour to meals. Or you could use smaller amounts of stronger tasting cheeses like Parmesan or strong Cheddar.
5. Reduce/eliminate meat and processed meat. Trim the fat off meat and skim it off the top of stews and gravies.

3 ways to get more omega 3s

1. If you struggle to source fresh fish, try canned fish, such as sardines, but opt for the type canned in water, as brine contains a lot of salt and omega 3s can be lost in oil.
2. Shellfish, such as fresh mussels and oysters, are good sources of omega 3, plus they are sustainable too.
3. Flaxseeds and walnuts are also good sources, although there are some questions about how readily the body can absorb plant forms of omega 3s.

Oils

Oils contain different percentages of saturated and unsaturated fats, making some healthier choices than others. Their suitability for cooking can depend on a combination of factors, such as antioxidant content, how they are produced and smoke point.

They can be produced in a variety of ways. At one end of the spectrum there are cold-pressed oils while at the other there are refined oils.

Extraction methods

Expeller-pressing
A mechanical, chemical-free extraction process, where the nut or seed is placed under pressure to extract the oil. No external heat is used during expeller pressing, but the temperature of this process will vary depending on the hardness of the seed or nut. The pressure that is needed for harder nuts or seeds causes more friction and heat.

Cold-pressing
An oil that has gone through the expeller pressing process while the temperature was controlled and kept below 50°C (122°F). Since the process does not involve an excess amount of heat or chemical solvents, cold-pressed oils maintain their original flavour and nutritional value as well as their antioxidant properties.

Refined oils
Extracted by using high temperatures and treated with chemical solvents that degrade their flavour, taste and nutritional composition.

This is why I choose cold-pressed oils wherever possible.

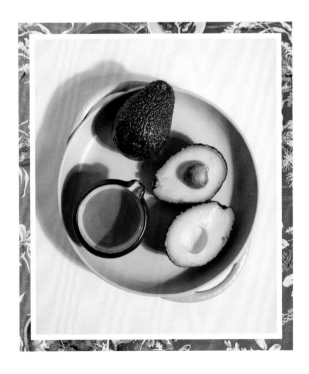

Types of oils

Extra virgin olive oil
Hands down the best oil. Research points towards the high antioxidant content of extra virgin olive oil providing protection when it is heated. So, cook with it (the good-quality stuff can take the heat of home cooking, up to 190°C/375°F), but also use it cold on salads, or to dip bread into.

Make sure you're getting the minimally processed stuff by looking out for the LOT number (a unique code that manufacturers assign to a batch of goods they've produced in the same run using the same ingredients, parts, or materials) and harvest date on the green bottle (the bottle should be green to prevent sun damage and preserve nutrients in the oil).

Rapeseed oil and sunflower oil
Despite high smoke points, both are high in omega-6 oils and oxidize easily when ground/pressed, so consequently have been linked to inflammation.

Coconut oil
This plant oil is primarily a saturated fat and has been found to raise LDL cholesterol, so is best used occasionally.

Butter
Primarily a saturated fat, so should therefore be limited, but it is also a source of vitamin A and contains calcium. Try to choose grass-fed organic butter if possible. (See page 20 for more information on grass fed/pasture fed.)

FACT CHECK

Is coconut oil good for me?

Coconut oil has been touted as a superfood with numerous health benefits. However, a lot of the hype, such as promoting weight loss or improving heart health, has no real science behind it. If you enjoy coconut oil then it's fine to include in small quantities as part of a balanced diet.

---

8 oil tips

1. Try to use sparingly, and preferably add on to food cold after the food has been cooked.
2. Try to avoid all refined oils. If the extraction is carried out by solvents, check the label to see the extraction method – if it doesn't say, it's likely solvents have been used.
3. Watch out for oils that are a blend of an expensive oil with a cheaper oil. Again you will need to check the label to see if this is the case.
4. Try to choose 100 per cent organic, extra virgin, cold-pressed or expeller pressed. Also by choosing organic you limit the amount of GMOs (genetically modified organisms) and hexanes, a chemical used in the extraction of oils.
5. Store your oils in dark, not clear, bottles away from light and heat, otherwise they turn rancid (rancidity creates free radicals that might increase your risk of developing diseases).
6. Don't store them on the kitchen counter or next to the stove.
7. Choose lids that close tightly and immediately store oil after using as if the oil gets too much exposure to oxygen it will go rancid.
8. Oils go bad over a span of months, depending on their type, which is why it's so important only to purchase the amount you'll use during a two-month period.

Action points

1.   Limit saturated fat
This mainly comes from animal sources such as
butter, cream, cheese, fatty meats and processed
meats, and are the dominant fat in some plant oils
such as coconut oil. See 5 ways to limit saturated
fats, page 39.

2.   Increase omega 3s
Some of the best foods for omega-3 fatty acids
are oily fish such as SMASH-T (salmon, mackerel,
anchovies, sardines herring and trout). The best
vegetarian sources of omega 3 are omega-3 eggs,
chia seeds and flaxseeds (try to buy these seeds
whole and grind them yourself as they oxidize
quickly once ground).

3.   Fall in love with extra virgin olive oil
Extra virgin olive oil is hands down the best oil.
Cook with it, but also use it cold on salads, or
dip bread into.

Try to choose 100 per cent organic, extra virgin,
cold-pressed or expeller-pressed minimally processed
oil by looking out for the LOT number and harvest
date on the green bottle (the bottle should be green to
prevent sun damage and preserve nutrients in the oil).

4.   Stay clear of trans fats
Research shows us that trans fats are linked to
bad health and heart disease, and are banned in
some countries. Refer to 5 ways to avoid artificial
trans fats on page 38.

Include fermented, prebiotic & probiotic foods

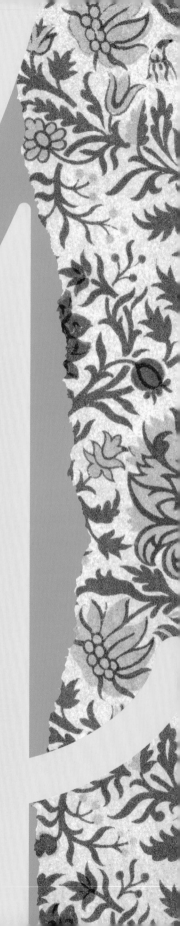

The key to a healthy functioning gut is the diversity of bacteria living in it.

We all have millions of bacteria, viruses, fungi and other organisms living in and around our body, mostly in our large intestine, which are also known as our gut microbiome. Current scientific thinking is that the microbiome is an entity in its own right, and not only do the microbes in it outnumber our genes but they are potentially just as influential. These microbes help to produce vitamins, control our blood sugar levels, manage hormones and cholesterol, control the calories we absorb and store, prevent us from getting infections, communicate with our nervous system and brain, and even influence our bone strength. Amazing, right?

What is the gut microbiome?

The gut microbiome is established in the first three years of our life, initially coming from our mother's birth canal and breastfeeding. Infants then acquire bacteria from their diet, environment and the people they interact with. As adults, our gut microbiome is strengthened or weakened by factors such as stress levels, sleep, diet and lifestyle choices.

No two people will have the same gut microbiome, not even identical twins – they are as unique as our fingerprints, except that they are always changing.

A diverse gut is a healthy gut. The greater the diversity of the different microbial species in the gut, the better, as a diverse gut microbiome is more likely to better withstand the environmental and biological challenges of daily life. Different bacteria respond to different foods, so what you choose to eat really does impact your microbiome. If you want to positively impact your gut microbiome, then one sure-fire way to do this is to consume high levels of fibre. Fibre is what the good bacteria feed off and what allows them to make short chain fatty acids (SCFAs). SCFAs affect how much energy we extract from what we eat and how we burn that energy. They also nourish the immune cells that line our gut and prevent damage and inflammation to the gut wall. They keep our blood sugar stable and modulate appetite.

It's never too late to start improving your gut health and the simple act of piling a more diverse range of plants on to your plate is enough to enhance your microbiome and transform your health (see pages 26–27).

Why the gut microbiome is so great

Microbes protect us. They are able to differentiate between harmful pathogens and harmless bacteria passing through the intestines, making them an important part of our immune system. They can also reshape and cultivate according to their environment and can swap genes and parts of DNA.

They also impact almost every aspect of our biology, from our ability to regulate appetite, break down food, make vitamins and absorb nutrients to producing or inhibiting serotonin production.

In addition, while the research is still very much in its infancy, the majority of it points towards gut-microbiome-driven inflammation being key in the development of attention deficit hyperactivity disorder (ADHD), Parkinson's and Alzheimer's disease, polycystic ovary syndrome (PCOS), diabetes, obesity, autism and autoimmune conditions, as well as influencing cardiovascular health.

What is dysbiosis?

Dysbiosis is a fancy way of saying your microbes are out of balance. The main reasons this occurs are:

1. Too much bacteria or overgrowth of unwanted elements.
2. Bacteria being in the wrong part of the gastrointestinal tract.
3. Lack of diversity, low numbers of certain bacteria or missing species.

What influences your gut microbes
— How you were born (natural birth or caesarean)
— Infant feeding (breast -ed or formula)
— Exercise
— Medication
— Diet
— Drugs, cigarettes and alcohol
— Genetics
— Stress
— Age
— Where you live in the world
— Where you travel

The gut and immunity

Over 70 per cent of our immunity is in our gut, with our gut bugs being one of the key educators of our immune system. The long-term health of our immune system is founded in the first few years of life and influenced by how we are born, nourished and the environment we grow up in. Immunity is not genetic but rather educated by our environment and our experiences, with much of this happening in the gut. Without gut microbes playing this vital role, we can develop serious food allergies. The essential day-to-day task of our immune system is to maintain a balance between reacting to things that might hurt us, identifying things that won't, as well as things we need like good germs. A diverse and healthy gut microbiome is a crucial part of this process. The gut microbiome teaches the immune cells that not all microbes are bad, which in turn affects the immune system throughout the entire body, influencing many aspects of health, such as our cancer surveillance system, our recovery from illness, and how we deal with inflammation, such as allergies or autoimmunity.

The gut and the brain

Over the last 20 years, the gut-brain axis has become one of the most widely researched areas in biology and the idea that the gut and the brain are two separate entities is now widely discredited. Microbes, the majority of which live in our gut, are known to have a significant impact on how our brain functions. We feed the microbes in our gut and, in turn, they produce the molecules our brain requires; it's a symbiotic and interdependent relationship.

The vagus nerve is the largest nerve in our body and connects our brain to our gut, running through all the major organs on the way. Specific bacterial strains have been shown to utilize vagus-nerve signalling to communicate with the brain and to alter behaviour. Additionally, short chain fatty acids, which are produced by the bacteria in the gut, have been shown to affect how our brain works. There is also a relationship between some of the body's major neurotransmitters and the gut. For instance, 95 per cent of your serotonin (your happy hormone) is produced by your gut microbes, and your gut microbes have the ability to increase receptors in your brain called GABA receptors, which means your brain can utilize more of this relaxing hormone.

The gut and sleep

There is a causal relationship between sleep and the gut. Our gut microbes impact our sleep and sleep impacts the ability of gut microbes to function. The neurotransmitters produced and released by gut microbes, such as serotonin and GABA, play a role in our sleep-wake cycle. While sleep impacts all areas of our health, including our gut.

Our gut microbes also have their own circadian rhythm and work differently at different times of the day. The research is still developing in this area but currently shows us that the better quality sleep you get, the better your cognitive function, and the greater the number of beneficial microbes in your gut.

7 secrets for a good night's sleep

1. Your morning routine is more important than your evening routine. It's easier to control when you wake up than when you go to sleep so make sure you get up at the same time every day.
2. Build sleepiness. Don't be afraid of feeling sleepy. It's good and it means you will sleep well that night.
3. Create a good opportunity for sleep, ideally prepare for for 7–8 hours.
4. If you can't get back to sleep after about 25 –30 minutes of lying in bed, get up and do a relaxing activity until you start feeling sleepy. Lying in bed for prolonged periods, hoping you'll finally fall asleep, isn't an effective sleep strategy, and it can make you feel anxious and frustrated. Your brain will also start to associate bed with being awake if you do anything in it besides sleeping or sex.

FACT CHECK

The gut is not the brain's 'serotonin factory'.

Neurons in the brain make their own neurotransmitters. Additionally, the serotonin produced in the gut cannot cross the blood-brain barrier, so it's improbable that gut serotonin directly influences brain function via the blood stream. The mechanism by which current research suggests it could affect the brain is through the gut-brain axis.

5. Don't overcompensate for not sleeping well by going to bed early or lying in.
6. Quality over quantity of sleep. A good night's sleep isn't just about how many hours of sleep you get, but also the quality of that sleep – in other words, how restful and restorative that sleep was.
7. The more you stress about lack of sleep, the worse your sleep will get. Don't overthink it. Give yourself a break.

The gut and exercise

Recent studies suggest that an increase in exercise can enhance the number of beneficial microbial species in the gut and affect how they function. Research points to the idea that the microbes in people who exercise regularly produce more short chain fatty acids, which helps keep your gut lining healthy and regulates your immune system (amongst other things), than in those who don't.

The evidence is by no means conclusive, but the overall consensus is that exercise is important for your gut. This doesn't mean going mad in the gym, but the body likes to move, so whether it's going for a walk, or hitting a class, make sure the exercise works for you.

The gut and skin

Research has long pointed to the relationship between skin and gut health. For example, rosacea is associated with small intestinal bacterial overgrowth (SIBO), and inflammatory skin conditions, such as psoriasis, are linked to inflammatory bowel disease (IBD).

While the science is not there yet as to the gut-skin interaction, it is clear that diet has a supportive and preventative role in the development of skin disease. Incorporating the following as part of a sustained eating pattern may support good skin health:

— Essential fatty acids, particularly omega 3s. Good sources of these are oily fish, such as SMASH-T (salmon, mackerel, anchovies, sardines, herring and trout). The best vegetarian sources of omega 3 are omega-3 eggs, chia seeds and flaxseeds (try to buy these seeds whole and grind them yourself and use immediately, or store in the fridge for up to a week as they oxidize quickly once ground).
— Vitamin C-rich foods, such as citrus fruits, bell peppers and cruciferous vegetables
— Vitamin E-rich foods, such as extra virgin olive oil, sunflower seeds and almonds
— Polyphenol-rich foods, such as berries, nuts, herbs and spices
— Carotenoid-rich foods, such as bell peppers, broccoli and carrots
— Minerals, such as selenium, copper and zinc found in nuts and seeds, dark leafy greens, wholegrains, oily fish and shellfish
— Fermented foods, yogurt or kefir, kimchi, sauerkraut, miso and tempeh and kombucha

The gut and hormones

Your gut and its bacteria make a lot of chemicals that affect brain function – for example serotonin, as discussed above. The gut also has a central role to play in hormone regulation and how much oestrogen is circulating in the body at one time. Your gut microbes produce the enzyme beta glucuronidase, a function of which is to break down oestrogen in the gut. If you don't have enough microbes producing this or if you're producing too much, oestrogen levels will be impacted, which in turn will affect bowel movements, bone turnover, body fat, metabolism and skin. Some symptoms of possible high oestrogen in women include; bloating, swelling and tenderness in your breasts, fibrocystic lumps in your breasts, decreased sex drive, irregular menstrual periods, increased symptoms of premenstrual syndrome (PMS), mood swings, headaches, anxiety and panic attacks, weight gain, hair loss, cold hands or feet, trouble sleeping, sleepiness or fatigue and memory problems.

What are fermented foods?

Fermented foods are defined as foods or beverages produced through controlled microbial growth, and the conversion of food components through enzymatic action. So, when bacteria and yeast 'pre-digest' food and drink, producing a range of vitamins, beneficial organic acids and other health-promoting compounds, this is fermentation. Generally, anything that uses microbes to transform simple ingredients is a 'fermented food'. Traditional fermented foods are associated with a whole host of potential health benefits, including:

— increasing vitamin concentrations (such as folate and vitamin B12)
— reducing anti-nutrients (which are substances that block or interfere with how your body absorbs other nutrients out of your gut and into your bloodstream)
— lowering blood pressure
— supporting immunity
— having a calming effect
— potentially lowering gluten in some sourdough bread and lactose content in some dairy

What are prebiotics?

Prebiotics are a specific type of fibre and the food for good bacteria, enabling them to thrive and work effectively. One of the best natural probiotics is called inulin, which boosts the number of bifidobacteria and which some studies have shown can help maintain the gut's mucus barrier and prevent inflammation.

A key benefit of prebiotic foods is that the different non-digestible fibres are broken down by the gut bacteria to produce short chain fatty acids. These SCFAs provide fuel for our gut lining, contribute to blood sugar balance, help things to move through the large intestine, support immunity, stimulate the release of gut hormones and directly impact fat tissue.

Some good sources of prebiotics are: onions (particularly good when eaten raw), garlic (particularly good when eaten raw), leeks, chicory root, asparagus, artichokes, olives, pulses and legumes, apples, pears, plums, wholegrains, such as 100 per cent rolled oats, nuts, such as almonds.

What are probiotics?

The World Health Organization defines a probiotic as a live microorganism which, when eaten or drunk in adequate amounts, confers a health benefit on the host. Probiotics can come in food or supplement form, and different strains will have different effects.

The three main criteria to fulfil the probiotic definition are:

1. The microbes have to be alive.
2. They have to be present in large numbers.
3. They have to have evidence of a health benefit.

There are a large selection of probiotic products, from probiotic-rich shot drinks (many of which contain quite a bit of sugar) to probiotic capsules. Overall, if you eat a healthy diet, you shouldn't require probiotic supplements.

A concern around probiotic food is how many microbes can survive the acidic conditions in the stomach in order to reach the colon intact and be able to colonize there.

Do all fermented foods contain probiotics?

No. Not all fermented foods contain live cultures, or use strains of microbes that have proven health benefits that can survive the trip through the gut. Additionally, not all fermented foods have adequate amounts of microbes to qualify as a probiotic. As listed above, there are a number of fermented 'probiotic' foods, but you should check the labels carefully to see what strains, if any, they contain. Additionally, live strains will be destroyed by processes like canning or pasteurizing so don't opt for these versions. You're far more likely to find probiotic-rich foods in the refrigerated section of the supermarket than the dried-good section of the supermarket.

Examples of fermented 'probiotic' foods

Yogurt (try to choose natural with no added sugar)
A dairy product made by fermenting milk with bacteria. Make sure you choose unflavoured options with 'live cultures' or 'live active bio cultures'. Quite often the good bacteria we want in the yogurt is killed off in the manufacturing process, so it's important to make sure you are buying a yogurt that still has it in, or has had it added back in. Try to mix up the brand or type of yogurt you buy as different yogurts contain different strains of bacteria (look at the label to see which ones each contains).

Kefir (try to choose natural with no added sugar)
A fermented milk or water using kefir grains to produce
a sour-tasting drink or yogurt. It's easy to make yourself
if you order the kefir grains, and you can flavour it with
lemon or different fruits. It is also widely available in
supermarkets now. Use it like yogurt. Kefir is a great
source of both pre- and probiotics. Again, try to make
sure you are going for options with 'live cultures' or
'live active bio cultures' in.

Kimchi
A traditional Korean side dish of salted and fermented
vegetables. It's delicious to have as a snack or works
well as a condiment. I love having it with eggs.

Sauerkraut
Sauerkraut is finely cut raw cabbage that has been
fermented by various lactic acid bacteria. If you're
buying it from a supermarket, look for unpasteurized
versions to make sure it still contains the good bacteria
and don't cook it before you eat it. Sauerkraut is
delicious on top of stews, in a sandwich or with a salad.

Miso
Miso is a traditional Japanese seasoning. It is
produced by fermenting soybeans with salt and
kōji and sometimes rice, barley, seaweed, or other
ingredients. It's great for creating dressings or
using as a marinade for vegetables, fish or meat.

Kombucha
Kombucha is a fermented, lightly effervescent,
sweetened black or green tea drink. It can be a
great alternative to alcohol. It's a bit of a faff to
make yourself, so if you're buying, opt for low-sugar
versions, as some can be quite sweet.

Note:
Live strains will be destroyed by heat-based processes
like canning or pasteurizing. So try to look for
unpasteurized jarred versions.

I try to include one of the above fermented foods in my
diet at least every day. It's usually kefir as I tend to have
that on my oats most mornings. I also buy kimchi (as
it's a bit of a fuss to make) and keep a jar in the fridge
for a quick and easy snack, or to eat alongside eggs.

Benefits of 'probiotic' foods

The research is still ongoing as to which strains
do what. There is some evidence to suggest that
probiotics are of benefit to relieve diarrhoea caused
by infection, gastroenteritis or allergies or after a
course of antibiotics. Additionally, certain strains
of probiotics have been found to reduce symptoms
of irritable bowel syndrome.

There is some limited research to suggest that
regular yogurt eaters have a reduced risk of type
2 diabetes, while consumption of kimchi has been
associated with a reduction in blood pressure and
insulin resistance.

There is also some additional research that points to
the idea that it's not just the bacteria in the fermented
foods that bring the benefits, but the fermentation
process actually predigests the food, making it easier
for our body to turn it into SCFAs.

The position you poo in matters

Emptying your bowels easily is an important part of good health. However, the 90-degree angle most of us in the Western world sit in to go to the toilet is not optimal for releasing our bowels. Squatting, on the other hand, where the knees are above the hips, allows the puborectalis muscle in the sphincter to relax and the rectum to open.

If you fancy giving this a go, you can either raise your knees up by putting your feet on a box or footstool/poop step (or you can use a waste paper bin) or lift up the loo seat and sit on the bowl of the toilet. This places you in a lower position, and consequently your knees will be higher in respect to your hips.

Sitting

Puborectalis muscle contracts, squeezing rectum. Increases straining and pelvic floor pressure.

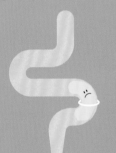

Squatting

Puborectalis muscle relaxes, allowing rectum to open. Prevents straining and protects nerves.

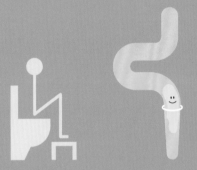

Action points

1. **Go whole and varied – no need to peel fruit and veg**
   Once again, whole foods and diversity are key to good gut health (see more on page 18).

2. **Eat probiotic and prebiotic foods**
   Refer to the list of probiotic- and prebiotic-rich foods on pages 47–48.

3. **Make sure you poo in the optimal way**
   Refer to the illustrations above.

*If you are pregnant, breastfeeding, have high histamine levels or are immunocompromized, fermented foods are not for you – seek advice from a medical professional.

Reduce
Refined
Carbohydrates

This is not a recommendation for a low-carb diet, as carbohydrates are essential for a healthy functioning body. Carbohydrates are found in most plant-based foods and play a valuable role in gut health by providing useful fibre to the digestive tract.

Our body breaks down carbohydrates into glucose. Glucose is the body's preferred source of energy, and is an essential fuel for the brain, aiding concentration. Carbohydrates also play an important role in generating the brain's serotonin supply (this is the happy hormone), so help to enhance mood. Serotonin is made from tryptophan and carbohydrates help convert tryptophan into serotonin. Serotonin is also converted into the hormone melatonin, which helps to regulate our circadian rhythm, so carbohydrates play a role in our sleep-wake cycle too.

What are refined carbs?

Refined carbs, also known as simple carbohydrates, include mostly sugars and processed grains. They can be a great source of quick energy, but lack essential nutrients and often contain unwanted additives, such as salt and hydrogenated fats. They include sugars and refined grains, such as white bread, pizza dough, pasta, pastries, white rice, sweets and desserts, as well as many commercially produced breakfast cereals, most of which have been stripped of their fibre and nutrients. Refined carbs are essentially calorie-rich but nutrient-poor. Carbohydrates in their natural state are nutrient-rich and fibre-rich and release energy much more slowly.

Refined carbs can also cause blood sugar to spike rapidly as they are often finely ground or dissolved in sugar and so are digested very quickly. A surge in blood sugar stimulates a surge in the hormone insulin, which brings our blood sugar rapidly back down and leaves us feeling hungry again. This can lead to a cycle of recurring hunger spikes, which isn't good for the body and can cause weight gain. If this goes on for too long, the body can also develop insulin resistance, which is when it stops responding to insulin, even when there are dangerously high levels in the blood. Insulin resistance is the main cause of type 2 diabetes.

Refined carbs have also been associated with a pro-inflammatory dietary pattern, which is linked to many diseases. Furthermore, diets high in refined carbs are associated with an increased risk of cancer, stroke and heart disease as they are known to raise triglycerides, cholesterol and blood pressure levels.

In essence, refined carbs offer empty calories, little in the way of nutrients and do not provide a feeling of satiety, often leaving us feeling hungry again not long after being consumed. They drive hunger and overeating, disrupt our blood sugar and energy levels, and are linked with a growing number of health conditions. When it comes to nutrition, I prefer to talk about all the wonderful things we can add into our diets as opposed to what we should take away. Unfortunately, refined carbohydrates are everywhere, and are heavily marketed, so it can be a challenge to avoid them, but the more whole foods we include in our diet the more these processed refined carbohydrates will naturally fall away.

The difference between simple (refined) and complex carbs

Carbs in their most basic form are monosaccharides (single-molecule carbohydrates).

Known as refined or simple carbs, they fall into three groups:

Glucose — Grains, pasta

Fructose — Fruit, veg, honey

Galactose — Dairy

When two molecules bond chemically, they form disaccharides, such as:

Lactose — Dairy

Sucrose — Sugar beet, cane sugar

Maltose — Molasses, beer

When multiple molecules bond together, they form polysaccharides. These complex carbs can be made up of hundreds, even thousands, of monosaccharides and include whole foods, such vegetables, beans, pulses and wholegrains.

What is the glycaemic index?

— The glycaemic index (GI) rates carbohydrates according to how quickly they raise the glucose level of the blood.
— The glycaemic load (GL) rates carbohydrates according to the glycaemic index and the amount of carbohydrate in the food.
— GL takes into account both GI and the amount of carbohydrate in the food. If a food is low GI, it does not mean you can eat a larger serving of that food – the total amount of carbohydrate and kilojoules eaten is still important.

For example, pasta has a lower GI than watermelon, but pasta has a higher GL than watermelon. So, if you eat the same amount of both, pasta will have the greater effect on your blood sugar levels.

FACT CHECK

Do carbs make you fat?

It's calories (rather than nutrients) that make a difference to weight. But this is only part of the story. If you're looking only at nutrients or calories, this misses the enormous complexity of what determines weight gain. Energy balance (and therefore body weight) is determined by a vast number of physiological, biological and social factors, some of which we can control and others we cannot.

What foods contain refined carbs?

Fizzy drinks, squashes and fruit drinks

Sweets and chocolates

Biscuits

White bread, including wraps, sandwiches and pizza

Ready meals

Lots of breakfast cereals

Crisps, tortilla chips and pretzels

Pastries, such as croissants

Ice cream

Cakes, muffins, scones and doughnuts

White pasta, white noodles and white couscous

Ketchups and sauces

Jams, honey and marmalade

Chocolate spread

Rice cakes

Sweetened yogurts and desserts

Some stock cubes

Some protein bars

Some veggie burgers

Some baby food

7 healthy swaps for refined carbs

1. Snack on nuts, seeds and dried fruit instead of grain snack bars as they come without the added sugar.
2. Swap milk chocolate for dark chocolate. Chocolate with 75 per cent cocoa solids content contains antioxidants, minerals and fibre as well as less sugar. Eat a square at a time and try pairing it with nuts and dried fruit to add extra nutritional bang.
3. Swap jams and marmalades for homemade stewed fruits made without additional sugar.
4. Eat better bread. Swap white bread for bread made with at least 50 per cent wholemeal flour and minimal additives. Ideally, the ingredients should be only yeast, salt, water and a small amount of fat/oil. Reducing the amount of bread you eat also allows more space in your diet for increasing the number of whole foods you eat.
5. Swap sugary breakfast cereals for oats.
6. Swap rice cakes for oat cakes or brown rice cakes.
7. Opt for natural yogurt and add fruit to it instead of having flavoured yogurt.

A note on sugar

There are two types of sugar – **non-free and free.** Non-free sugar is sugar naturally contained within the cell structure of food and is found in fruit and vegetables, starchy carbohydrates, grains and dairy products. Because these sugars are contained within the cell wall, our bodies need to work harder to release them, which means they don't cause such high elevations in blood sugar levels.

Any form of added sugar is considered a free sugar. Free sugars are often added to baked goods but can also be released from the cell structure during processing – for example, when fruit is turned into fruit juice. Just like refined carbs, refined sugars – white, golden, brown, coconut sugar, maple syrup, agave and honey – are absorbed very quickly by the body.

Try to avoid high fructose corn syrup (HFCS), which is packaged into many foods in the US. HFCS has been linked to diabetes, reduced insulin sensitivity, increased risk of developing high blood pressure and high cholesterol levels.

Sugar intake recommendations

The World Health Organization (WHO) recommends that no more than 5 per cent of our daily energy intake come from free sugar. In the UK, recommendations are to limit sugar to no more than 90g (3¼oz) per day and for no more than 30g (1oz) of that to be free sugar. Try to become aware of how much sugar you're consuming and where it's coming from, so you can stay within the limits and make better food choices.

7 ways to reduce sugar consumption

1. Sugary drinks in particular have been linked with weight gain and a number of health problems. Try swapping sugar-sweetened beverages (fizzy drinks, sweetened juice, squash and cordial) for fizzy or still water, fruit-flavoured water or cold brew teas, herbal teas, broths and soups.
2. Try swapping sugary foods, such as biscuits, for oat cakes with some nut butter on and, instead of a sugary breakfast cereal, add real fruit to oats.
3. Try to scale back or avoid adding sugar into food when cooking.
4. Shop-bought biscuits and cakes are one of the biggest culprits when trying to reduce sugar consumption. While these items are not something to consume every day, if you can't fathom a life without them, then consider making them yourself. Swap white flour for wholegrain, reduce the amount of sugar in the recipe by as much as your taste buds allow (I go for a 50 per cent reduction). Think about substituting in whole foods, such as nuts, dried fruits, fruits or

vegetables. Also, remembering that these items are a treat and not something for everyday will help too.
5. Swap sugary breakfast cereals for 100 per cent rolled whole oats, avoid instant/quick oats
6. Condiments such as ketchup can have 22g (⅘oz) of sugar per 100g (3½oz), so try to use smaller servings
   or an alternative, such as mustard.
7. Reduce and then remove sugar in hot drinks. For example, just 1 teaspoon of sugar in your tea can add up to 16g of sugar in one day if you drink four cups of tea, which is over half your daily sugar allowance. Try drinking liquorice tea instead when a sugar craving strikes.

Some people can give up sugar immediately, but others need time to adapt. There has not been enough research into this so there is no prescription as to the amount of sugar-free days needed to reset your palate. A majority of people find that three days of total cold turkey (including sugar from fruits and juices) is enough to recalibrate their palate enough so that they can taste the natural sugars in food more. Tastebuds undergo continual turnover and their average lifespan has been estimated as approximately 10 days, which may also provide a good timeframe for people to aim for. But the truth is it can take time to retrain your palate, so if at first you don't feel like it's working, keep going! Eventually everything will catch up.

7 tips to help reduce sugar cravings

1. Sleep. Aim to get your 7–9 hours of sleep every night and try not to use your phone for at least 30 minutes before bedtime.
2. De-stress. Managing stress and anxiety is important. Try some simple relaxation techniques to help relieve stress, such as breathing, meditation or yoga.
3. Mindful eating. A number of studies highlight the benefits of mindful eating in managing food cravings, so try removing distractions while you eat and turning it into a mindful experience.
4. Avoid 'cutting out' craved foods. There's no need to completely eliminate foods, and the chances are you will crave them more if you do.

5. Switch it up. If your cravings are bothering you, try to mix up when you eat certain foods to break 'conditioned' habits, such as going for a daily walk when you'd usually crave a sweet treat mid-afternoon. Lots of my clients report that drinking liquorice tea when they are getting a sugar craving helps to manage them.

6. Enjoy it! Looking after your health is about inclusion, not restriction. Balance and diversity is key, so don't beat yourself up for 'giving in' to cravings. Enjoy everything in moderation and think about adding in some plant-based foods with whatever you're eating.

7. Get rid of the guilt. If having some chocolate before your period makes you feel good, don't feel guilty about it.

Why it's important to read the label!

A lot of the refined carbs we eat are hidden in processed foods, so it's useful to be able to spot them on the label – look for less added sugar, low salt and more fibre from wholegrains. Refer to page 15 for more information on sugar.

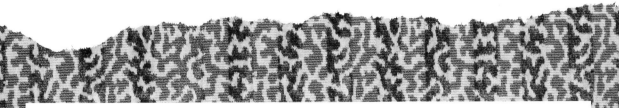

Action points

1. **Focus on consuming quality carbs**
   Learning which carbs are beneficial for health and which are less so is invaluable to enjoying a healthier diet. Unrefined carbs are full of fibre and nutrients that are beneficial to our health. Refined carbs are the opposite, they have had all the goodness stripped out and are just empty calories. So, wherever possible, cut back on refined carbs and opt for whole food options instead.

2. **Reduce sugar consumption**
   Sugar alone is not responsible for the refined carb problem, but it can be a quick and easy one to act on. Limit consumption of sugary foods, particularly those high in free sugars, and try to avoid adding sugar to food items yourself. Refer to '7 ways to reduce sugar consumption' on page the opposite page.

3. **Read labels**
   Get to grips with what it is you are consuming, and particularly try to limit items with a high free sugar content. Or even better, opt for as many whole foods as possible, and cook from scratch when you can, then you won't have to worry about what ingredients are in your food!

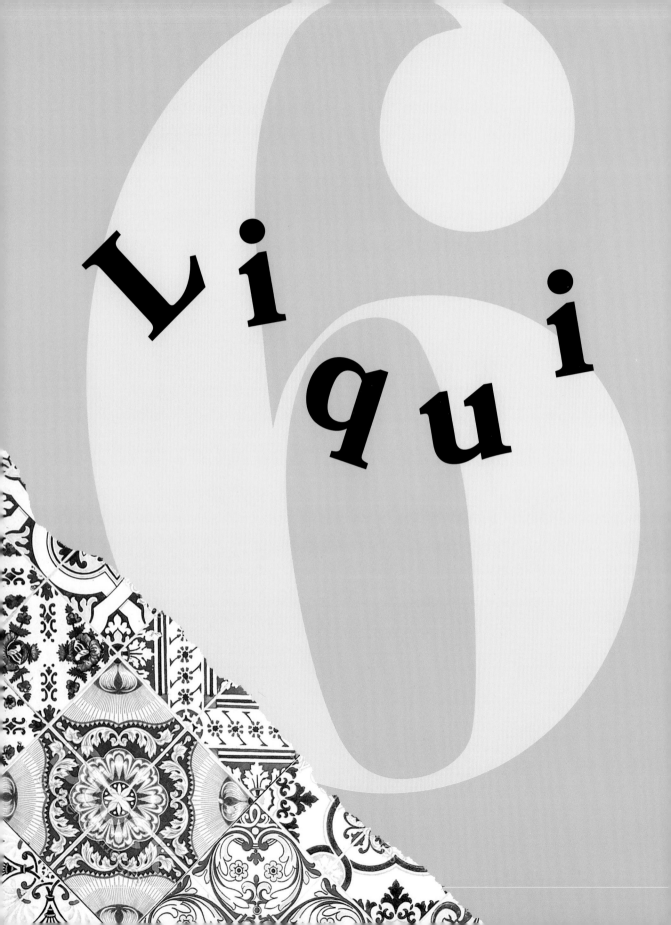

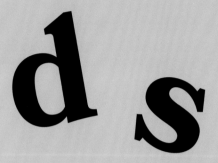

Hydration is a crucial part of nutrition but one that is regularly overlooked. Water is essential for all the body's processes to work, a point that is illustrated by the fact that we can survive much longer without food than we can without water.

Our circulatory system needs water for blood to flow around our body, delivering vital nutrients to our cells. Our brain is 75 per cent water and needs water to carry out essential functions. Our kidneys need water to filter out waste products. Our digestive system needs water to help break down the food we eat, allowing nutrients to be absorbed by the body. Our body is constantly losing water each day, so it is vital that we frequently replace it.

How much water should we be drinking?

The UK Eatwell Guide and the NHS recommend that we drink 1.2–1.6 litres (42–56fl oz) of water every day. This equates to 6–8 glasses of 200ml (7fl oz) a day. The European Food Safety Authority (EFSA) suggests an adequate total daily intake of 2 litres of fluids for women and 2.5 litres for men. This quantity includes drinking water, drinks of all kinds and the moisture available from the food we eat. On average, our food is thought to contribute about 20 per cent of our fluid intake which, therefore, suggests a woman should aim to drink about 1.6 litres and a man should aim for 2 litres. In the US, the National Academy of Medicine suggests an adequate intake of daily fluids of about 9 cups (2.1 litres) and 13 cups (3.1 litres) for healthy women and men, respectively, with 1 cup equalling 8 ounces (this includes water from foods). These targets may also need to be adapted, depending on your lifestyle and environment, so if you exercise or are in a hot country, for example, you will need to drink more water.

Signs of dehydration

Dehydration has a negative effect on mental and physical functioning, which becomes more severe as dehydration increases. Symptoms of dehydration in adults and children include:

— feeling thirsty
— dark yellow and strong-smelling pee
— feeling dizzy or lightheaded
— feeling tired
— a dry mouth, lips and eyes
— peeing little, and fewer than 4 times a day

Urine colour check

The best guide to how well you are hydrated is the colour of your urine. Check out the chart below to see where you sit.

Calculate your water needs

This is a general calculation that can help you work out your daily water requirement. You may need to make adjustments depending on your activity and environment, but the general rule is:

Your weight in kg x 0.033 = the litres of water per day you should drink

So if someone weights 60kg, this would mean they need to be consuming 1.98 litres a day.

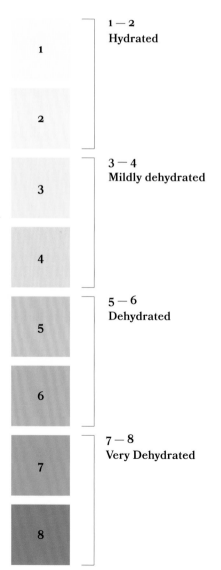

1 — 2
Hydrated

3 — 4
Mildly dehydrated

5 — 6
Dehydrated

7 — 8
Very Dehydrated

Tips to drink more water

— Keep a glass of water beside your bed and where you work.
— Buy a reusable water bottle to keep in your bag or car for when you go out.
— Flavour your water with fruits, vegetables, or cold brew teas.

Calorific drinks

Our brain does not recognize drinking calories in the same way as eating calories – when we eat calories our body responds very differently to when we drink them. When we eat calories, the brain sends out signals that it is full and to stop eating, but if we drink the same number of calories, our brain tells the body it is still hungry.

Also, when we chew our food our body releases hormones to tell us we are eating, but when we don't chew, we don't release these hormones, so the brain doesn't know it's getting fed. Additionally, the longer it takes for food to pass through the digestive system, the more satisfying it is. Calorific drinks shoot through the digestive system without filling us up but leave loads of calories behind. It can be helpful, therefore, to think of these drinks as food, not drinks.

Sugar-sweetened beverages (SSBs)

SSBs are fizzy drinks, such as cola, energy drinks, sports drinks, squash and fruit-flavoured drinks and waters. They are some of the biggest sources of unwanted sugar in our diets. A 340ml (11½fl oz) can of cola, for example, contains an average of 39g (1½oz) of sugar, which is more than the daily recommend allowance in one drink!

SSBs don't fill us up and they can actually drive hunger, so they are terrible for weight gain, plus they are associated with the accumulation of dangerous visceral fat around the internal organs, increased blood pressure and an increased risk of type 2 diabetes. They can also drive inflammation, which contributes to many chronic diseases.

7 tips to help you cut out SSBs

— Buy a reusable water bottle to keep in your bag or car for when you go out.
— Identify when you are most likely to reach for a sweet drink and try to pre-empt that by doing something else that is less triggering, like going on a walk or playing a game.
— Instead of having an SSB, have a glass of water first instead. You might just be thirsty so it could stop the craving entirely.
— Have a small snack, such as a handful of nuts or an oatcake with peanut butter on; this could help to balance your blood sugar, which may be triggering the craving.
— Have a cup of unsweetened tea, plain coffee or liquorice tea, as this helps to quell the sweet craving.
— Try diluting the SSB down with still or fizzy water.
— Try cold brew teas or herbal teas for a caffeine-free alternative.

Fruit juice and smoothies

The latest UK guidance is that even freshly pressed juices and homemade smoothies should be limited to one 150ml (5fl oz) serving a day. You might wonder why, given that they are made from whole food ingredients with no additives. Well, the juicing or blending process changes the structure of the fruit, altering the way our body responds to it. The natural sugars in the juice, when pressed or blended, become free sugars, and our body reacts to them in much in the same way they do the sugars in SSBs. As explained in Principle 5, free sugars are sugars that are not contained within the cell structure of food and so are absorbed extremely quickly into the body.

On the plus side, juices and smoothies do contain some nutrients (such as vitamins and minerals), unlike SSBs which have no nutritional value, but if you want to make a smoothie, it's best to leave fruits with edible skins unpeeled (to increase their nutrient value) and not to over-blend them, as this will reduce the amount of free sugars. Unless otherwise advised by a health-care professional, it's probably best not to opt for juicing or blending your vegetables over eating them whole entirely. However, using liquified veggies to supplement your diet definitely has its benefits.

Caffeine

Tea and coffee are amongst the world's most popular beverages (obviously!), and for most people, when consumed in moderation, the caffeine in them is beneficial rather than harmful. As well as creating a welcome ritual, drinking tea and coffee can give us a quick energy boost and increase alertness.

Tea and coffee are also rich in antioxidants, which protect our bodies against free radical damage and may help prevent the development of certain chronic diseases, such as cancer and cardiovascular disease. Tea and coffee are not the best source of antioxidants, but it does mean that if you are wedded to your cup of tea of coffee, then you don't have to give it up.

The general guidance therefore is that moderate caffeine intake, around 300–400mg per day, which equals 3–4 cups of coffee, or five mugs of tea, can have beneficial effects. More than 600mg caffeine daily, however, can cause insomnia, nervousness, irritability, increased blood pressure and an upset stomach, although response to caffeine varies hugely from person to person, so it's important to listen to your body and know your right level.

The danger lurking in your high-street coffee

Café culture has brought with it a significant health problem, which is that the traditional coffee with a bit of milk has been replaced with calorie-laden lattes, cappuccinos, cream-topped mochas, with syrups and sugars added in. What was a 20–40-calorie drink can now pass the 500-calorie mark. As we've already learned, these calorific drinks shoot through the digestive system without filling us up but leave significant calories behind.

FACT CHECK

Does caffeine give you energy?

Caffeine doesn't literally give you energy as it doesn't contain any calories. It makes you feel more awake by stimulating your nervous system and can possibly improve your mood. It is thought that caffeine blocks receptors in the brain that promote sleepiness, and other receptors in the brain which, when blocked, produce dopamine (a 'feel good' neurotransmitter, which plays a role in body functions including movement, memory, motivation and reward).

Caffeine sources

Hot chocolate
5mg, 1oz

Milk Chocolate
5mg, 1oz

Dark Chocolate
15mg, 1oz

Soda
30–40mg, 12oz

Green/black tea
30–50mg, 8oz

Black coffee
80–100mg, 8oz

Energy Shot
200mg, 0.2oz

Pure caffeine
Extremely potent

Alcohol

While you may not want to give alcohol up completely, it is good to limit your alcohol intake. UK Health guidelines state that adults should not regularly drink more than 14 units of alcohol per week and ideally less. Please refer to page 31 for more information on individual countries drinking guidance. For optimal gut health, we should drink none.

Heavy prolonged drinking can lead to the development of chronic diseases and other serious problems, including high blood pressure, heart disease, stroke, liver disease and digestive problems. Alcohol has also been linked to several cancers and is classed as a group 1 carcinogen.

Alcohol is dehydrating. It causes the body to remove fluids from the blood through our renal system, which includes the kidneys, ureters and bladder, at a much quicker rate than other liquids. If you don't drink enough water with alcohol, you can become dehydrated quickly.

Alcohol can also increase the amount of acid in our stomach. This can irritate the stomach lining and cause indigestion and heartburn.

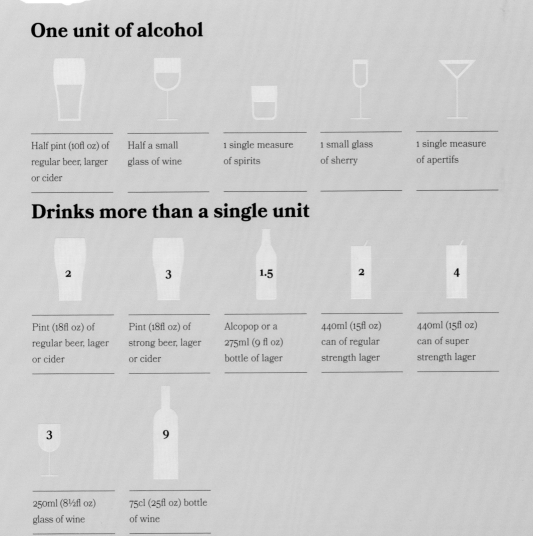

One unit of alcohol

Half pint (10fl oz) of regular beer, larger or cider

Half a small glass of wine

1 single measure of spirits

1 small glass of sherry

1 single measure of apertifs

Drinks more than a single unit

2 Pint (18fl oz) of regular beer, lager or cider

3 Pint (18fl oz) of strong beer, lager or cider

1.5 Alcopop or a 275ml (9 fl oz) bottle of lager

2 440ml (15fl oz) can of regular strength lager

4 440ml (15fl oz) can of super strength lager

3 250ml (8½fl oz) glass of wine

9 75cl (25fl oz) bottle of wine

Alcohol is a sedative, so it can initially make it easier to fall asleep, but as the night progresses it can create an imbalance between slow-wave sleep and REM sleep, resulting in poorer quality sleep.

Alcohol is also packed full of calories. A large glass of wine or a pint of beer each carry around 200 calories. Alcohol also tends to encourage us to make poor food choices and eat more than we would when not intoxicated.

Drinking pattern is also important. Research suggests that people who drink a little, spread over more days, have a lower death rate than those consuming the same amount over 1–2 days. So, a little spread out over a few days is better than a lot consumed in a short amount of time, but I would still recommend trying to have several alcohol-free days a week.

How many calories are in your drink?

Beer 4% 1 pint (568ml)	183 calories
Red wine 12% 175ml (6oz) glass	147 calories
White wine 12% 175ml (6oz) glass	147 calories
Spirits 40% single (25ml/0.8oz)	61 calories
Champagne 12% 125ml (4oz) glass	89 calories
Martini 90ml (3oz)	165 calories
Cosmopolitan 120ml (4oz)	244 calories
Margarita 120ml (4oz)	168 calories
Manhattan 120ml (4oz)	187 calories
Pina Colada 260ml (9oz)	490 calories

How to deal with a hangover

The only real cure to avoiding a hangover is to drink moderately – or not at all! – but there are ways you can bounce back and avoid being stuck in bed the entire day. And none of them involve mythical hangover cures,

such as eating fried foods or having more to drink the following day, which obviously isn't a good idea. It's worth bearing in mind that the severity of a hangover has a lot to do with your nutrient status before you start drinking, particularly your levels of vitamin B3 and zinc. Having a meal of foods rich in these, such as salmon with quinoa, or prawns and brown rice, will stand you in good stead. Once you have your hangover, these things will help:

— Drink an electrolyte-, potassium-rich beverage, such as coconut water.
— Suck on a ginger candy, have some ginger tea or chop up some ginger and add it to yogurt or a smoothie.
— Eat a well-balanced breakfast. Focus on high-nutrient, hydrating foods and high-quality protein, such as oily fish, beans and legumes.
— Sweat it out. Doing a workout will release endorphins in your body as well as speed up your metabolism so you can process the alcohol quicker.
— Go easy on the caffeine. Coffee is a diuretic, which can enhance dehydration, so be sure to consume it alongside a glass of water.
— Have a nap as alcohol can cause broken or disrupted sleep.

Going alcohol-free

Now more than ever we are questioning what we are putting in our body, and the impact it is having on our physical and mental health. We know alcohol disturbs our gut microflora and sleep, plus it contributes to anxiety and depression, so it's no surprise it has come into the firing line.

If you're sober curious, you're not alone. There are a growing number of people who are interested in the benefits of not drinking alcohol. Choosing to go sober doesn't have to be a reaction to being physically dependent on alcohol or realizing it is ruining your life. It can just be about a feeling that alcohol is taking away more from your life than it is adding in. So if you're bored of wasting days being hungover or worrying about what you've said, done or texted the night before, then these tips could help.

9 ways to make going alcohol-free easier

1. Join alcohol-free Instagram accounts and Facebook groups. There's a lot of support on these forums as well as inspiration and motivation.

2. Talk to your friends about it. If you tell people you're going alcohol-free, you'll find it easier to keep to your resolution and they can help support you.

3. Arrange activities that lend themselves to being alcohol-free more easily – play a sport, organize a movie night, go hiking, sign up to an evening class, enjoy a games night.

4. Be prepared – if you're going somewhere where you know people will be drinking, work out in advance what you will drink instead of alcohol. Non-alcoholic beer can taste just as good as the original and is a great option if you don't feel like drawing attention to the fact you're not drinking. Also look out for non-alcoholic wines and cocktails as these are becoming more and more readily available.

5. Make the most of hangover-free mornings. This could involve cooking, making breakfast plans with friends, or learning a new skill, or exercise.

6. Listen to sobriety podcasts or read a sobriety book.

7. Take an online course on how to stop drinking.

8. Download a sober app.

9. Join an organization that helps people stop drinking. This is also an opportunity to meet new sober friends.

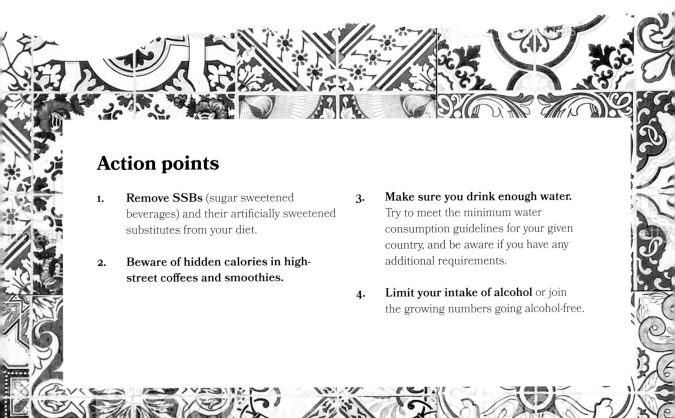

Action points

1. **Remove SSBs** (sugar sweetened beverages) and their artificially sweetened substitutes from your diet.

2. **Beware of hidden calories in high-street coffees and smoothies.**

3. **Make sure you drink enough water.** Try to meet the minimum water consumption guidelines for your given country, and be aware if you have any additional requirements.

4. **Limit your intake of alcohol** or join the growing numbers going alcohol-free.

Eat Mindfully

For many of us, mealtimes are rushed affairs. We can find ourselves mindlessly shovelling down food without thinking, either while we are commuting, sat in front of a computer screen at work or on the sofa at home watching TV. Eating while doing something else is a very disconnected way to consume food and frequently results in us finishing our food without even noticing we have eaten it. Often, we eat for reasons that have little to do with hunger and more to do with emotion, such as to relieve stress, or to cope with boredom, loneliness, sadness or anxiety. Paying attention to the experience of eating, however, can improve your diet, manage food cravings and even help you to lose weight.

Eating food and absorbing food are also two very different things. The digestive process starts with the act of preparing food, and the smells and colours alert our body to the fact that it needs to start preparing for digestion, so we salivate and start producing digestive enzymes. If we remove this part of the digestive process, we are failing to maximize the benefits we can get from the food we are eating.

What is mindful eating?

Mindful eating is about paying attention to how you feel as you eat and drink, the texture and tastes of each mouthful, as well as your body's hunger and fullness cues, and how different foods affect your energy and mood. It has little to do with calories, carbohydrates, fat or protein. The purpose is not to lose weight, although those who adopt this style of eating regularly do, but rather to savour the moment and the food and be aware of the eating experience. It requires us to acknowledge and accept, rather than judge, these feelings, thoughts and bodily sensations.

Mindful eating isn't about calorie counting, restriction, eating the 'right' things, being perfect or never eating on-the-go again. Rather, mindful eating focuses all your senses on being present when you shop, cook, serve and eat your food. Eating in this way, even for just a few meals a week, can help you become more attuned to your body. It can also make it easier to implement better dietary habits and enjoy the improved well-being that comes from them, as well as help to prevent overeating.

The benefits of mindful eating

Although the research is still developing in this area, mindful eating appears to offer numerous psychological and physical health advantages such as helping us:

— Understand our body's hunger, craving and fullness cues
— Develop a better relationship with food
— Eat only when we're hungry
— Allow food cravings to pass
— End a meal when we're full
— Stop binge eating
— Stop emotional eating
— Lose weight
— Promote heart health
— Control blood sugar
— Promote healthier responses to stress
— Increase the variety of food we eat
— Spend less time thinking about food
— Slow down and take a break from the hustle and bustle of our day, easing stress and anxiety
— Make healthier choices about what we eat
— Improve our digestion by eating slower
— Feel fuller sooner and by eating less food

How to eat mindfully

1. **Start with your shopping list.** Consider the nutritional value of every item you add to your list and try and stick to it to avoid impulse buys.

2. **Eat with an appetite, but not when super hungry.** Missing meals can often lead to wanting to stuff anything in your mouth later on in the day so you end up not really thinking about the quality of what you are eating or enjoying your food.

3. **Sit at a kitchen/dining table to eat.** Don't eat hunched over on the sofa or in front of a computer screen.

4. **Start with a small portion – you can always come back for more.** Limiting the size of your plate to 23cm (9in) or less and using a smaller knife and fork can help to reduce the speed at which you eat and the volume of food you consume.

5. **Appreciate your food.** Before you start eating take four deep breaths in through the nose and out through the mouth. Or pause for a minute or two before you begin eating to contemplate everything and everyone it took to bring the meal to your table. Be thankful for the opportunity to enjoy delicious food and the people you're enjoying it with.

6. **Be aware.** Bring all your senses to the meal, so pay attention when you're cooking, serving and eating your food. Be attentive to colour, texture, aroma and even the sounds different foods make as you prepare them. As you chew your food, try identifying all the ingredients, especially seasonings.

7. **Small bites.** Don't overfill your fork. Maybe try eating with a smaller knife and fork and from a smaller plate.

8. **Slow down.** Try putting your knife and fork down between mouthfuls.

9. **Chew each mouthful.** Depending on what you are eating try to chew each mouthful at least 15 times for softer foods like bananas and 30 times for tougher foods like steak. Really try to taste your food.

For most of us, the idea that we can be mindful of every mouthful of food we take or every meal we eat is unrealistic. Many are faced with their only option being to eat on the move or not eat at all. But the good news is, you don't necessarily have to stick to a full mindfulness eating routine in order to avoid eating mindlessly or ignoring your body's hunger or fullness cues.

Consider whether you're eating in response to hunger cues or to an emotional signal. Maybe you're bored, lonely, sad or anxious? In which case you will need to address the underlying driving factors behind why you feel like that. Question whether you're eating food that is good nutritionally or that is emotionally comforting. If you must eat at your desk, are you able to take a few moments to focus all your attention on your food, rather than be distracted by a computer or phone?

Every little bit of mindful eating counts. The more you can do to slow down, focus solely on the process of eating and listen to your body, the more satisfaction you'll get from your food and the better nutrition habits you'll be able to establish.

Mindless eating

Eating highly processed, junk or comfort food

Eating without thinking or while doing something else (driving, working, reading, watching TV, etc.)

Emotional eating (because you're bored, stressed, sad, lonely)

Eating food as quickly as possible

Eating until all the food has gone, ignoring your body's fullness cues

Mindful eating

Eating nutritionally valuable food

Focusing all your attention on your food and the experience of eating it

Eating only to satisfy physical hunger

Eating slowly, appreciating each bite

Listening to your body's fullness cues and eating only until you're full

Using mindfulness to explore your relationship with food

Hopefully, now you're on Principle 7, you will know that you should be aiming to eat a variety of whole foods and less sugar and refined carbohydrates. However, if simply knowing these principles of healthy eating was enough, no one would be overweight or addicted to junk food. Mindful eating is a missing part of the puzzle. When you eat mindfully you become more in tune with your body, and can start to feel how different foods affect you physically, mentally and emotionally. This makes it much easier to motivate yourself to make better food choices. For example, once you realize that the salty pizza you crave is a result of your hangover or the sugary snack you can't resist when you're tired or depressed actually leaves you feeling worse, it's easier to manage these cravings and go for healthier options that boost your energy and mood instead.

How does your food make you feel?

It's important to become aware of how different foods make us feel, not just after we swallow, but after 5 minutes, an hour, or several hours, and generally throughout the day.

To start tracking the relationship between what you eat and how it makes you feel, try the following exercise:

1. **Eat how you would normally.** Choose the foods, quantities and the times for eating that you normally would, only now add mindfulness when you are doing it.
2. **Pay attention to how you feel,** both physically and emotionally, 5 minutes after you have eaten, an hour after you have eaten and several hours after you've eaten. Has there been a shift or change as the result of eating? Do you feel energetic or sleepy? Do you feel better or worse?
3. **Record everything you eat and how you feel,** including snacks between meals. Make sure to write everything down as you go or track it in an app, you really won't remember it all otherwise!

Experimenting with eating habits

Once you're able to connect your food choices to your physical and mental well-being, the process of selecting food becomes a matter of listening to your own body. For example, you may find that when you consume carbohydrates you feel heavy and sluggish for hours. If so, you might try switching to wholegrains and including more protein with each meal. Different foods will affect us all differently, according to factors such as genetics and lifestyle, so it may involve some trial and error to find the foods and combinations that work best for you. The below exercise can help you discover how different food combinations and quantities affect how you feel:

1. Change the times you eat at. Try eating within a smaller window of hours during the day, having three meals evenly spaced throughout the day, or three meals with two snacks.
2. If you're a meat-eater, trial two or three days without meat in your diet.
3. Exclude red meat and include only chicken and fish.
4. Remove certain foods from your diet, such as salt, sugar, coffee or highly processed foods, and see if this affects how you feel.
5. Trial different food combinations. Try eating solely starch meals, protein meals, fruit meals or vegetable meals.

Record everything you notice in yourself as you experiment with your eating habits. The question you're trying to answer is: Which eating patterns make me feel better, and which make me feel worse?

Keep trialling different types, combinations and amounts of food for two or three weeks, tracking how you feel mentally, physically and emotionally. Everyone is different, so you are going to be the best person to decide what works for you and what doesn't. Once you learn to listen to your body, you'll become empowered with the knowledge of what it needs.

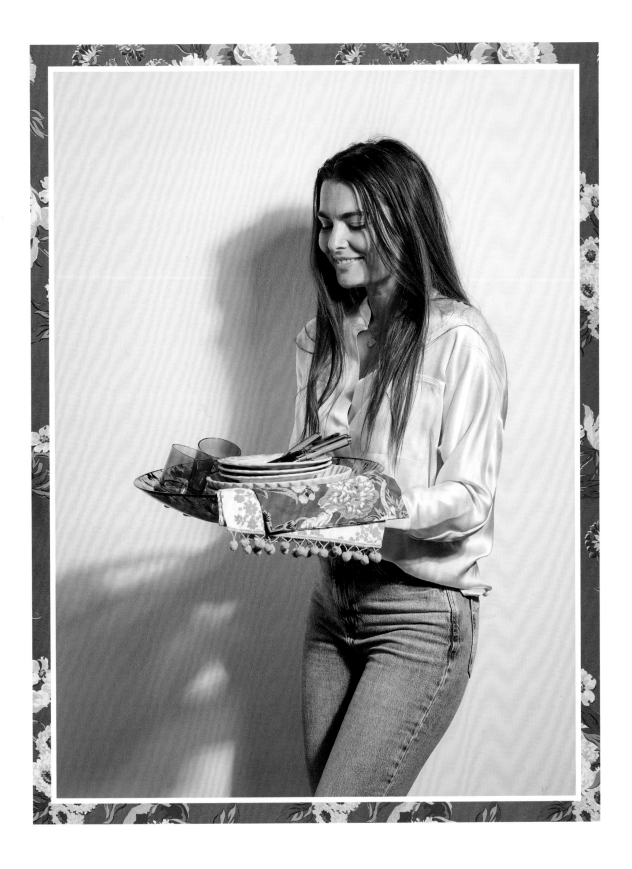

8 ways to fit mindful eating into real life

Starting to eat mindfully can seem challenging at first. You're changing the habit of a lifetime after all. So here are some suggestions to start you on your way...

1. **Don't overfill your plate.** How you fill your plate is an important consideration, so be aware of portion sizes when constructing a meal (see Principle 1, page 13). The idea of a carbohydrate base is now an outdated one and a more helpful way of approaching how you construct your plate is to start with the vegetables, ideally filling half the plate with them, then add a quarter of a plate with carbohydrate, ideally a wholegrain or whole food, then fill a quarter of the plate with a lean protein. Resist the urge to pile your plate high. You can always come back for seconds, and the act of delaying tends to help you eat less, as your body has more time to register its fullness.

2. **Love your leftovers.** Thinking more about portion sizes might mean cooking less. However, if you do cook more than you need relish, the fact that if you have leftovers, they can be the next day's lunch, rather than feeling you need to finish everything off.

3. **Question pre-packaged portion sizes.** Portion sizes have been slowly creeping up over the decades, so if you are eating pre-packaged foods (but hopefully you will be opting for mostly home-cooked meals!) be aware that what has been decided by the manufacturer might not be right for you. If the portion size is too big, for example, or doesn't contain enough vegetables, don't be scared to either halve it and/or add more vegetables.

4. **Be savvy when eating out.** I find that few restaurants serve meals containing enough vegetables, so when eating out you'll often have to think about the principles of how to construct an ideal plate and try to apply them to your order. It's not necessary, for example, to follow a restaurant's set menu – I frequently have two starters as a main, or a starter and then share a main with a side of vegetables.

5. **Takeaway tips.** Again, don't be scared to reset portions. If items come in a container, then decant them onto a plate to help you register the portion size. Eating straight from the container makes it much harder to gauge the amount. It's a good idea to try and reduce consumption of these anyway as takeaways often have added salt for flavour and preservation and are cooked in significant amounts of fat, as well as having sugar added to entice us into eating more of them.

6. **Keep a food journal.** Tracking what you're eating by writing down everything you consume can help you be more mindful about what you choose to eat. Often, we forget what we've just eaten, so it can be useful to reflect on our overall dietary picture. My clients are often surprised at how their diet looks when they see it all written down, and it can have a positive influence on their food choices and portion sizes.

7. **Don't reach for the sweet.** If, when you've finished eating, you find yourself reaching for something sweet, try resisting for 10 minutes. You may find the impulse has passed once this time is up. Making and drinking a cup of tea during this time can also help curb the craving. If you do still feel like something sweet, a square or two of dark chocolate is the best option.

8. **Avoid grazing.** It's good practice to have breaks between when you consume food, and not graze all day. Digesting food is an energetically costly and inflammatory process. If you snack all day long, this places an extra burden on your digestive system, whereas limiting your food intake to three times a day or to three times a day with two snacks means your body has time to recover in the periods between meals, which also means it is better able to digest the food when you do consume it. It's helpful to eat at similar times each day as well.

Intermittent fasting (IF)

Intermittent fasting (IF) is an eating pattern that cycles between periods of fasting and eating. Most IF diets don't specify which foods you should eat, but rather when you should eat them. The most common are:

— 16/8 Method – skipping breakfast and restricting when you eat to a period of 8 hours, such as 1–9pm.
— Eat-Stop-Eat – fasting for 24 hours, twice a week, by not eating from dinner one day until dinner the next day.
— 5:2 Diet – consuming 500–600 calories on two non-consecutive days of the week and eating normally for the other 5 days.

Everyone is different, so you have to find what method works best for you, but good general dietary advice is to limit food intake to a 10–12-hour window to allow your gut time to heal and repair. So, if you eat breakfast at 8am, then aim to have your last meal by 8pm.

Benefits of intermittent fasting

The main benefit of IF is weight loss, although no more so than with any other conventional calorie-restricted dieting approach. However, fasting has also been shown to improve certain risk factors, such as insulin sensitivity, which has implications for diabetes risk. Additionally, several studies have shown that fasting seems to promote greater efficiency at dealing with fat after a meal, which is an important cardiovascular disease risk factor. Having said that, the diabetic therapeutic benefits of fasting need to be closely monitored due to the risk of low blood sugars.

FACT CHECK

Does when you eat matter?

There is no conclusive evidence telling us when the best time of day to eat is. What does seem to play the most important role is routine. So calories eaten late at night won't automatically turn to fat, but avoiding skipping meals and eating at regular times throughout the day will help keep your body happy.

Action points

1. Before you start eating take four deep breaths. In through the nose and out through the mouth.

2. Sit at a table to eat, not hunched over on the couch.

3. When you are eating, try to just do that. Focus on chewing and eating your food and avoid watching TV or looking at your phone.

4. Put down your knife and fork between mouthfuls.

5. Be aware of portion sizes. Use smaller plates and cutlery.

6. Listen to your body, let it tell you when it is full.

7. Give yourself a break between meals and be consistent with eating times.

Breakfast & Brunch

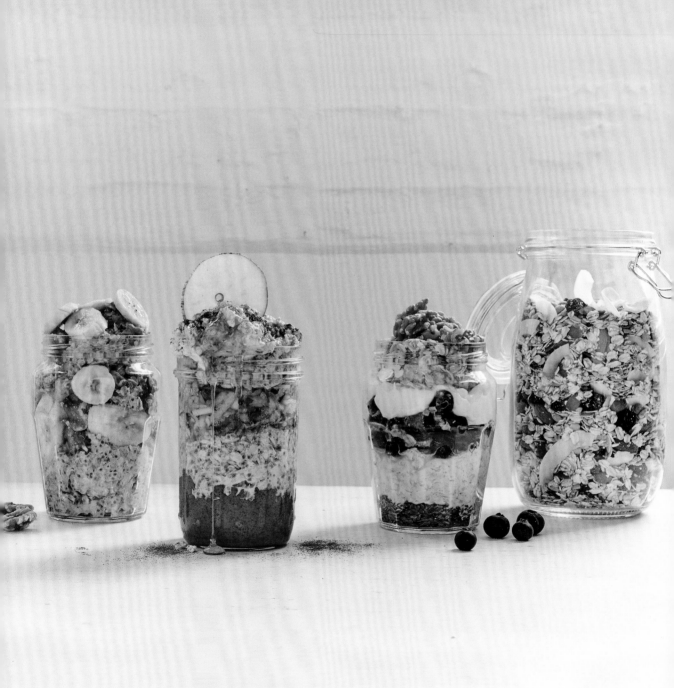

Speedy breakfasts

Banana and walnut oats Serves 1

40g (½ cup) 100 per cent rolled oats

175ml (¾ cup) almond milk

2 teaspoons chia seeds

1 banana, mashed

75g (½ cup) blueberries

½ tsp ground cinnamon

palm-sized serving of walnuts, roughly chopped

Combine all the ingredients in a bowl, then place in your chosen container. Pop in the fridge overnight to thicken or eat right away, if you prefer.

Easy apple pie porridge Serves 1

40g (½ cup) 100 per cent rolled oats

½ tablespoon chia seeds

½ teaspoon ground cinnamon

240ml (1 cup) almond milk

1 apple, cored and grated with skin on, plus extra to serve (optional)

1 teaspoon raisins

nut butter, to serve

Combine all the ingredients in a bowl and eat immediately or leave in the fridge to thicken overnight. When you're ready to serve, top with more apple and nut butter if you like.

Super-speedy breakfast Serves 1

40g (½ cup) 100 per cent rolled oats

185ml (¾ cup) almond milk

60ml (¼ cup) natural yogurt or kefir

1 tablespoon freshly ground flaxseed

palm-sized serving of walnuts, roughly chopped

150g (1 cup) blueberries

Combine all the ingredients in a bowl, then place in your chosen container. Pop in the fridge overnight to thicken or eat right away, if you prefer.

Muesli Makes about 6 portions

240g (3 cups) 100 per cent rolled oats

50g (½ cup) coconut flakes

80g (½ cup) raisins

30g (¼ cup) pumpkin seeds

150g (1 cup) almonds

30g (¼ cup) sunflower seeds

Place everything in an airtight container and shake to combine. When you're ready to serve, top with milk of your choice and fresh fruit. Store in an airtight container for up to a month.

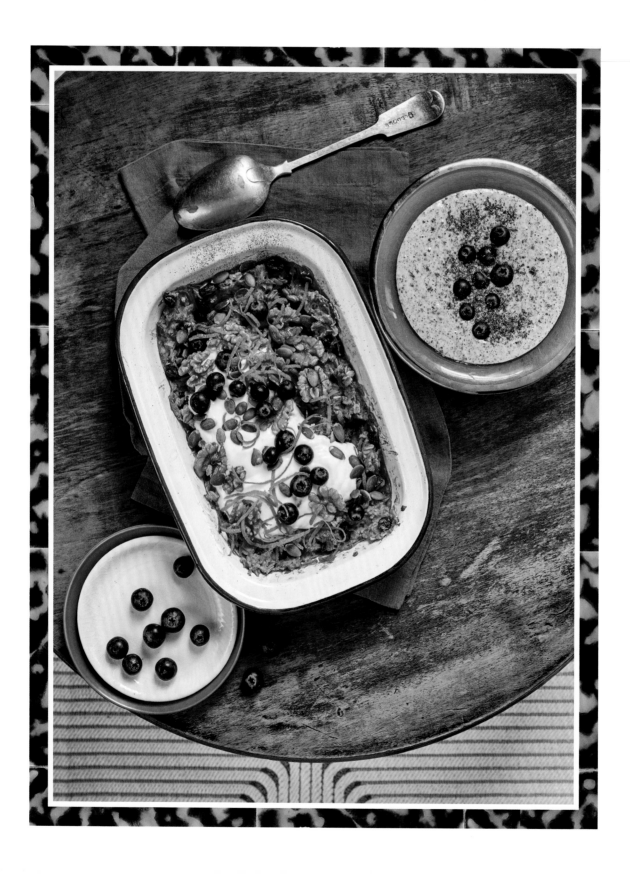

Flaxseed pudding Serves 1

Ingredients

3 tablespoons freshly ground flaxseed

150ml (5fl oz) plant-based milk

1 banana, roughly broken into pieces

1 date, pitted

fruits and berries of your choice, to serve

Method

1. In a bowl, cover the freshly ground flaxseed with the milk and put in the fridge to soak for at least 4 hours, or overnight if possible.

2. The following morning, transfer the flaxseed and milk into a blender cup with the banana and dates and blitz until smooth.

3. Serve topped with your favourite fruits or berries.

Carrot cake porridge bake Serves 1

Ingredients

extra virgin olive oil or coconut oil, for greasing

50g (1¾oz) 100 per cent rolled oats

½ carrot, scrubbed and grated

230ml (8fl oz) any kind of milk (I like almond milk)

½ teaspoon vanilla extract

½ teaspoon ground cinnamon

½ teaspoon nutmeg

pinch of salt

1 heaped tablespoon raisins (optional)

Toppings

yogurt

honey or maple syrup

pumpkin seeds

walnuts

orange zest

blueberries

Method

1. Preheat the oven to 200°C/180°C fan/400°F/gas mark 6 and grease a small ovenproof dish or ramekin with extra virgin olive oil or coconut oil.

2. Mix all the ingredients together in a bowl, then transfer to the prepared dish and bake for 25 minutes or so until golden at the edges.

3. Leave to cool for 10 minutes or so, then dollop with yogurt and a little honey or maple syrup and some pumpkin seeds, walnuts, orange zest and blueberries if you like. Enjoy straight from the dish.

Turmeric porridge Serves 1

Ingredients

40g (½ cup) 100 per cent rolled oats

240ml (1 cup) coconut milk

½ tsp ground turmeric

¼ tsp ground ginger

1 tsp ground cinnamon

1 tsp honey or maple syrup (optional)

Toppings

toasted flaked almond slices

fresh fruit (I like blueberries)

natural yogurt

Method

1. Add the oats and coconut milk to a pan over a medium heat and cook for about 5 minutes, or until bubbling.

2. Add the spices and stir frequently. If it gets too dry, add more coconut milk or a little water.

3. Finally, add the honey or maple syrup if desired.

4. Toast the almond slices in a small dry saucepan until they turn slightly golden brown.

5. Pour the turmeric porridge into a bowl and garnish with the blueberries, almond slices and a dollop of yogurt.

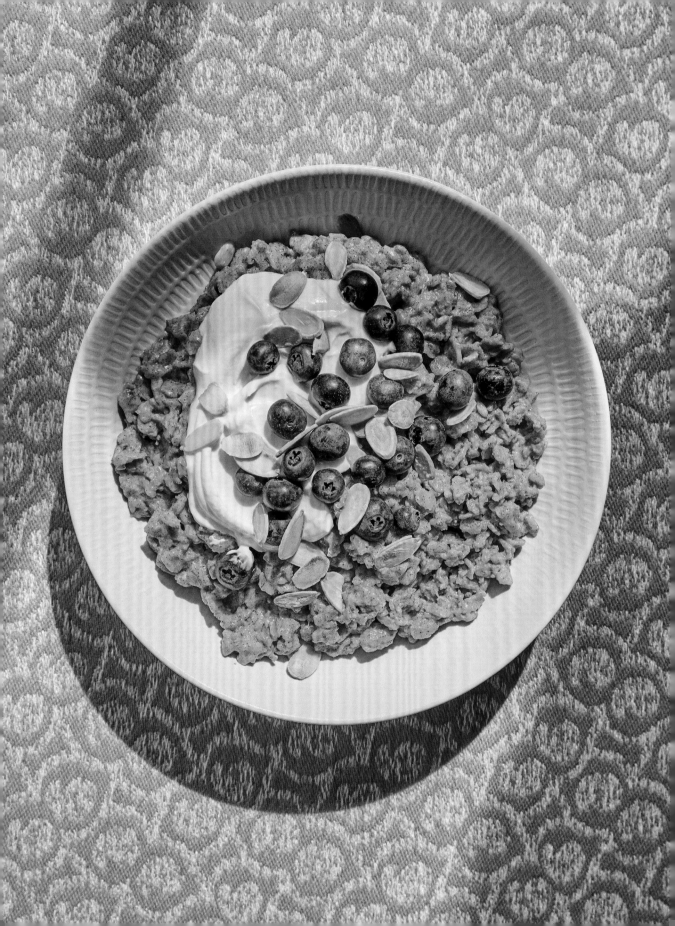

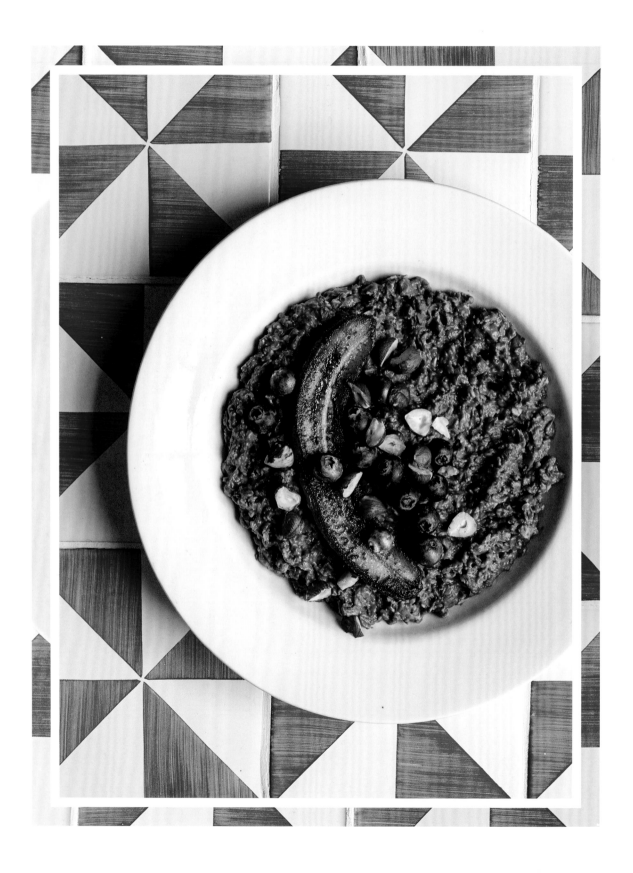

Chocolate banoffee porridge Serves 1

Ingredients

1 ripe banana

40g (½ cup) 100 per cent rolled oats

240ml (1 cup) any kind of milk (I like almond milk)

1 teaspoon cacao powder

1 tablespoon your choice of chopped nuts (I like hazelnuts)

1 tablespoon freshly ground flaxseed

1 handful of blueberries

maple syrup, to serve

Method

1. Mash one half of the banana in a bowl. Slice the remaining half and set aside.

2. Place a pan over a medium heat and add the oats, milk, cacao powder, mashed banana, chopped nuts and flaxseed.

3. Cook for 3–5 minutes until it reaches your desired consistency, adding more milk if you like it runnier.

4. Pour the porridge into a bowl and top with the sliced banana, blueberries and maple syrup. Enjoy!

Raspberry chia pudding Serves 1

Ingredients

120ml (½ cup) yogurt
or dairy alternative

120ml (½ cup) almond milk

35g (¼ cup) chia seeds

125g (1 cup) raspberries

Method

1. Mix the yogurt, almond milk and chia seeds together then decant into your chosen container (I use a small water glass). Then pop in the fridge for at least 2 hours, or overnight to thicken.

2. Once you're ready to serve, blend the raspberries (with a small amount of water if needed) until smooth.

3. Pour the blended raspberries onto the chia mixture in the glass, then enjoy!

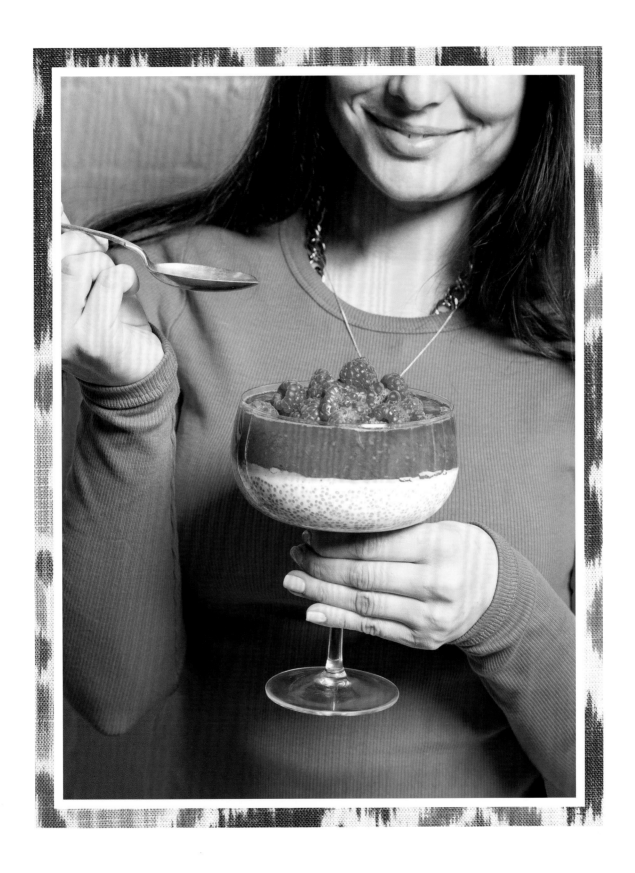

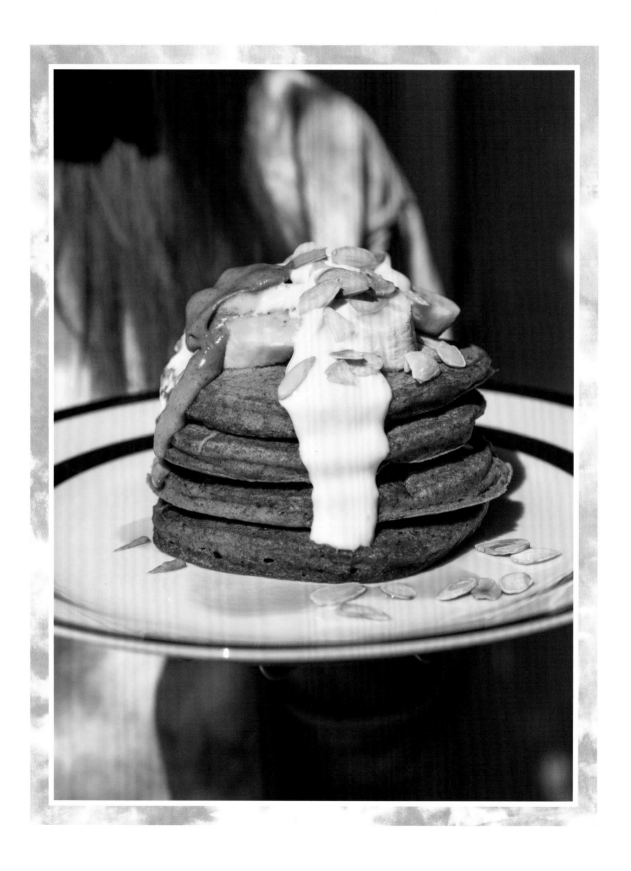

Spinach banana pancakes

Serves 1 (makes about 5 pancakes)

Ingredients

1–2 bananas

2 large handfuls of spinach

320ml (1⅓ cups) plant-based milk

280g (10oz) flour (I like buckwheat flour)

1 teaspoon bicarbonate of soda

½ teaspoon salt

extra virgin olive oil, for frying

Toppings
(optional)

nut butter

coconut yogurt

chopped banana

maple syrup or honey

Method

1. Blitz the banana, spinach and milk in a food processor or blender until smooth.

2. Pour the batter into a bowl and stir in the flour, bicarbonate of soda and salt until everything is combined.

3. Place a pan over a medium heat and add some extra virgin olive oil.

4. Pour in a ladleful of the batter to make a pancake about 10cm (4in) wide and 1cm (½in) thick and cook for about 5 minutes on each side until golden brown. Repeat with the remaining batter.

5. Add your favourite toppings; I went with peanut butter, coconut yogurt, chopped banana and maple syrup.

Mushroom shakshuka Serves 2–4

Ingredients

extra virgin olive oil,
for frying

1 medium onion, diced

1 red pepper, sliced

2 portobello mushrooms
(or you can use any
mushrooms you like), sliced

4 small tomatoes, cubed

4 garlic cloves, crushed

1 teaspoon paprika

400g (14oz) can plum tomatoes

1 tbsp za'atar

1 tablespoon freshly chopped
flat-leaf parsley, plus extra
to serve

2 large handfuls of
spinach, washed

4 organic free-range eggs

1 small handful of basil,
chopped, to serve

salt and pepper

Dressing

6 tablespoons natural yogurt

zest and juice of 1 lemon

2 garlic cloves, crushed

Method

1. Preheat the oven to 190°C/170°C fan/375°F/gas mark 5.

2. Heat some extra virgin olive oil in a large pan. Add the onion, red pepper, mushrooms and tomatoes and sauté over a medium heat for about 5 minutes until they begin to soften.

3. Add the garlic, salt, pepper and paprika and fry for a further minute.

4. Tip in the canned tomatoes, za'atar and parsley and simmer for around 10 minutes.

5. Place some spinach on top and allow to wilt.

6. Make four indentations in the tomato mixture and gently crack an egg into each one.

7. Place in the oven to cook for 8–10 minutes, or until the eggs are just set. Check regularly towards the end to make sure the eggs do not overcook.

8. While the eggs are cooking, place all your lemon yogurt dressing ingredients in a bowl over a pan of simmering water and cook, stirring regularly for 5–8 minutes.

9. Once your eggs are cooked, serve your shakshuka in bowls, drizzled with the lemon yogurt dressing and scattered with fresh basil and parsley. This goes very well with slices of sourdough bread to dunk in. Enjoy!

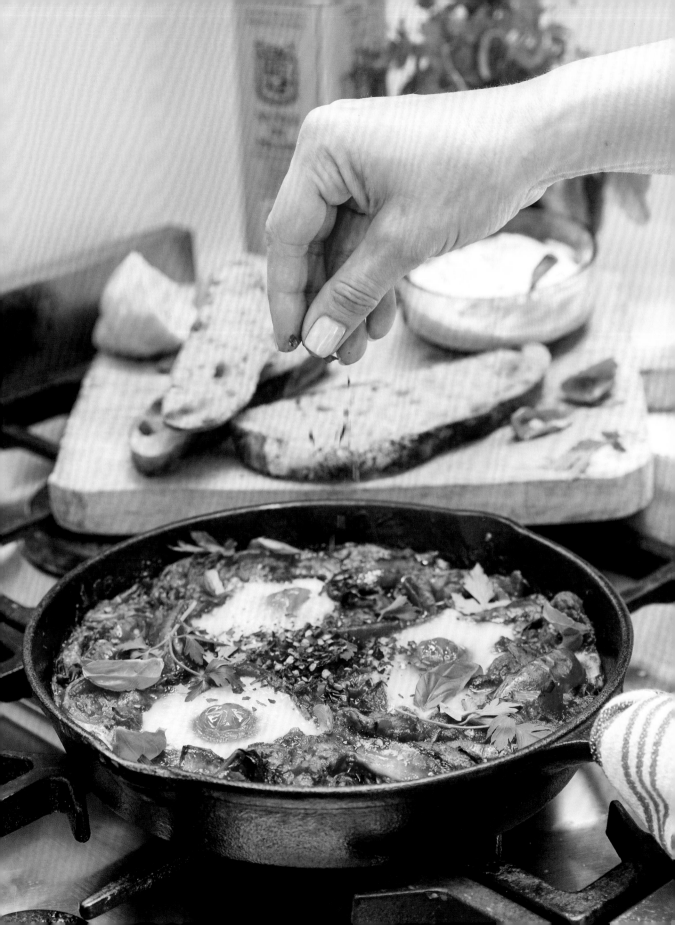

Sun-dried tomato butter beans on toast Serves 2

Ingredients

extra virgin olive oil, for frying

1 shallot, diced

120g (4¼oz) mushrooms
(I used closed-cup chestnut
mushrooms), sliced

1 garlic clove, sliced

400g (14oz) can butter beans,
drained and rinsed

120g (4¼oz) baby plum tomatoes

2 tablespoons sun-dried
tomato paste

½ teaspoon chilli flakes

80g (2¾oz) coconut yogurt

salt and pepper

2–4 slices brown or
sourdough toast, to serve

Method

1. Place the extra virgin olive oil in a pan over a medium heat and cook the shallot and mushrooms for 4–5 minutes, then add the garlic and cook for 1 minute.

2. Add the beans, tomatoes, sun-dried tomato paste, chilli flakes and yogurt to the pan. Season with salt and pepper and simmer for 4–5 minutes until the beans have heated through and the sauce has thickened.

3. Serve on top of warm brown or sourdough toast.

Cottage cheese toast with avocado Serves 1

Ingredients

2 slices of wholewheat
or sourdough bread

½ avocado

lemon juice

4 tablespoons cottage cheese

extra virgin olive oil,
for drizzling

freshly chopped dill (optional)

chilli flakes (optional)

mixed seeds (I use a mixture
of sunflower, pumpkin and
sesame seeds – optional)

salt and pepper (optional)

Method

1. Toast your bread in the toaster or under a hot grill.

2. In a small bowl, roughly mash the avocado and add a squeeze of lemon juice.

3. Spread the cheese onto the toast.

4. Spread the avocado on top of the cheese, then drizzle over some extra virgin olive oil and top with lemon juice, dill, chilli flakes, mixed seeds and salt and pepper if you like.

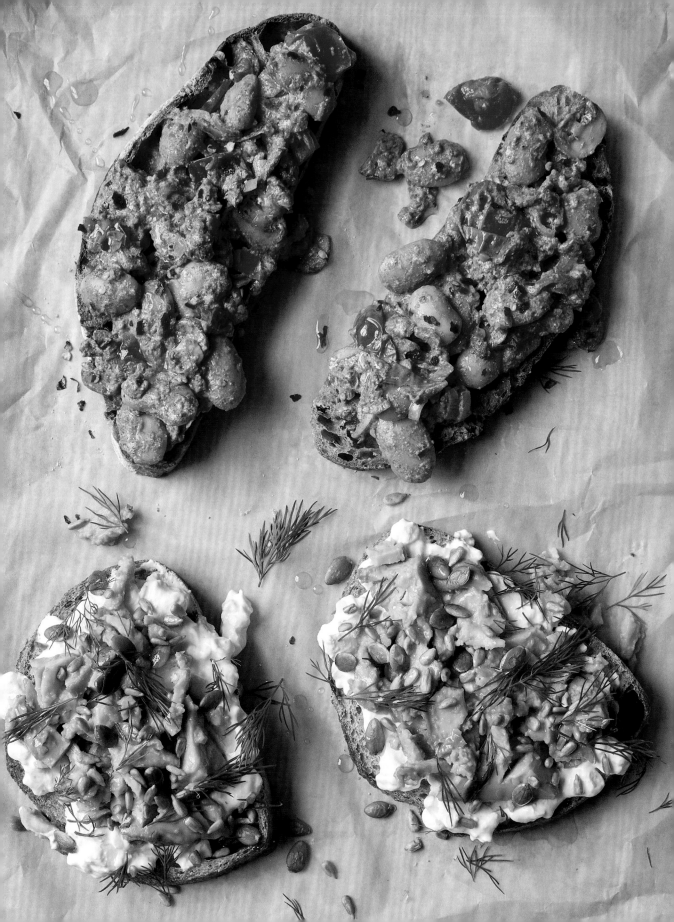

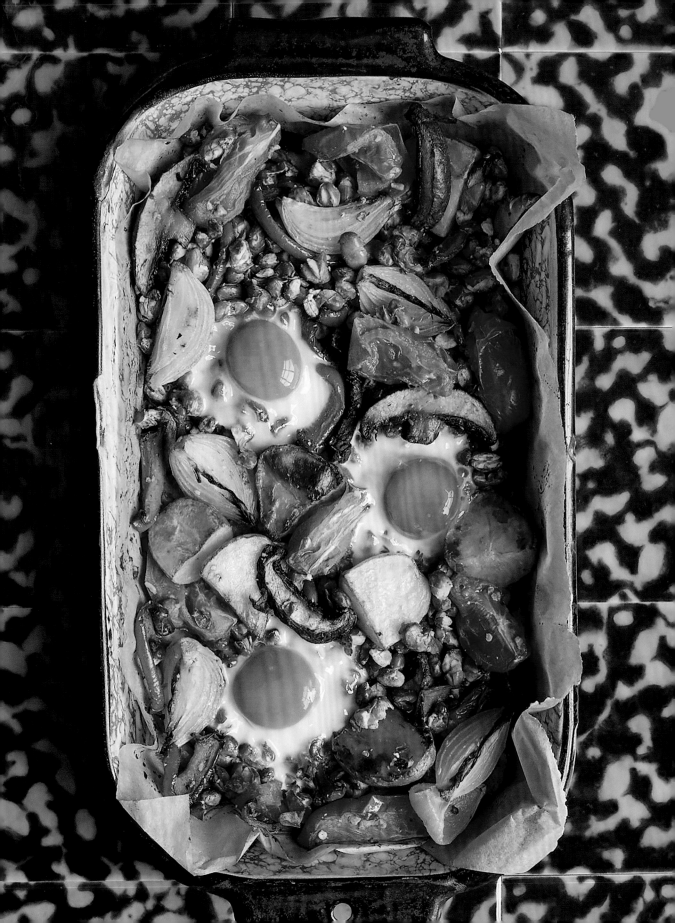

Loaded breakfast hash Serves 2

Ingredients

1 potato, cut into about 2cm (¾in) cubes

extra virgin olive oil, for drizzling

1 medium onion, sliced

1 red chilli, diced

2 medium tomatoes, quartered

1 green pepper, sliced

100g (3½oz) mushrooms (I used large portobello mushrooms), sliced

4 garlic cloves, crushed

400g (14oz) can pinto beans, drained and rinsed

1 tablespoon paprika

1 teaspoon chilli flakes

4 organic free-range eggs

salt and pepper

To serve

snipped chives

lemon juice

natural yogurt or coconut yogurt

avocado, sliced

Method

1. Preheat the oven to 180°C/160°C fan/350°F/gas mark 4. Spread out the potato on a lined baking sheet and cook for 10 minutes, then drizzle with extra virgin olive oil and cook for another 10 minutes until crispy.

2. Meanwhile, place the onion, chilli, tomatoes, green pepper, mushrooms, garlic and beans in a bowl and coat with extra virgin olive oil, and sprinkle over the paprika, the chilli flakes and some salt and pepper.

3. Onc the potatoes have baked, remove them from the oven and transfer to a pan along with the bean mixture, making sure everything is evenly spread out.

4. Bake in the oven for a further 15 minutes, or until everything has softened and just started to brown.

5. Give the mixture a good stir and make four little wells, then crack an egg into each of them. Pop the dish back in the oven for 8 minutes for soft eggs.

6. Top with chives, lemon juice, yogurt of your choice and avocado.

Soups
Salads
&
Sandwiches

Thai red curry noodle soup Serves 2–3

Ingredients

240g (8½oz) skinless chicken breasts or 300g (10½oz) tofu, cut into 2.5cm (1in) chunks

1 tablespoon extra virgin olive oil

1 onion, diced

3 garlic cloves, minced

3 tablespoons Thai red curry paste (how much curry paste you use will depend on which curry paste you use, so taste before adding)

1 tablespoon freshly grated ginger

700ml (3 cups) vegetable or chicken broth

400ml (14fl oz) can coconut milk

1 red pepper, diced

1 courgette, cut into semicircles

2 large handfuls of spinach

120g (4½oz) rice noodles

1 tablespoon fish sauce

salt and pepper

Toppings

4 spring onions, thinly sliced

fresh coriander leaves

fresh lime juice

Method

1. If you're using chicken, bring a pan of water to the boil and add the chicken breasts. Cook for 15 minutes, then remove from the water and use two forks to shred the chicken. Set aside.

2. Meanwhile, heat some extra virgin olive oil in a large pan over a medium heat. Add the onion and tofu (if using) and cook until the onion is translucent and the tofu has started to brown, about 4 minutes. Then add the garlic and cook, stirring occasionally, for about 1 minute.

3. Stir in the red curry paste and ginger and cook until fragrant, about 1 minute.

4. Stir in the broth and coconut milk. Bring to the boil, then reduce the heat and simmer for about 10 minutes, stirring occasionally, until reduced.

5. Add the red pepper and courgette, and cook for 5 minutes.

6. Next, add the chicken (if using), spinach, rice noodles and fish sauce, give everything a good stir and bring to a simmer. Cook for about 5 minutes until the noodles are tender.

7. Remove from the heat and top with the spring onions and coriander. Squeeze over the lime juice and season with salt and pepper, to taste. Then you're ready to serve.

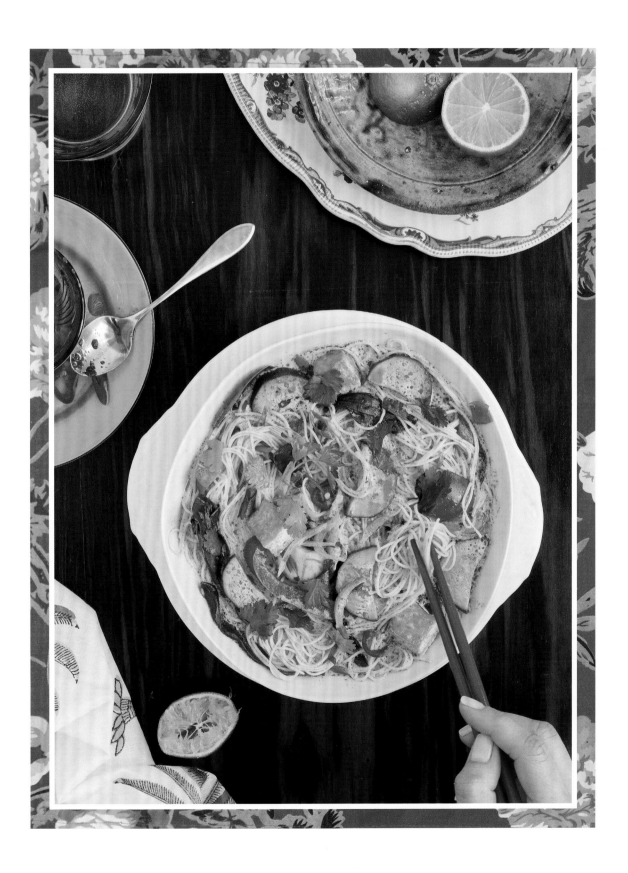

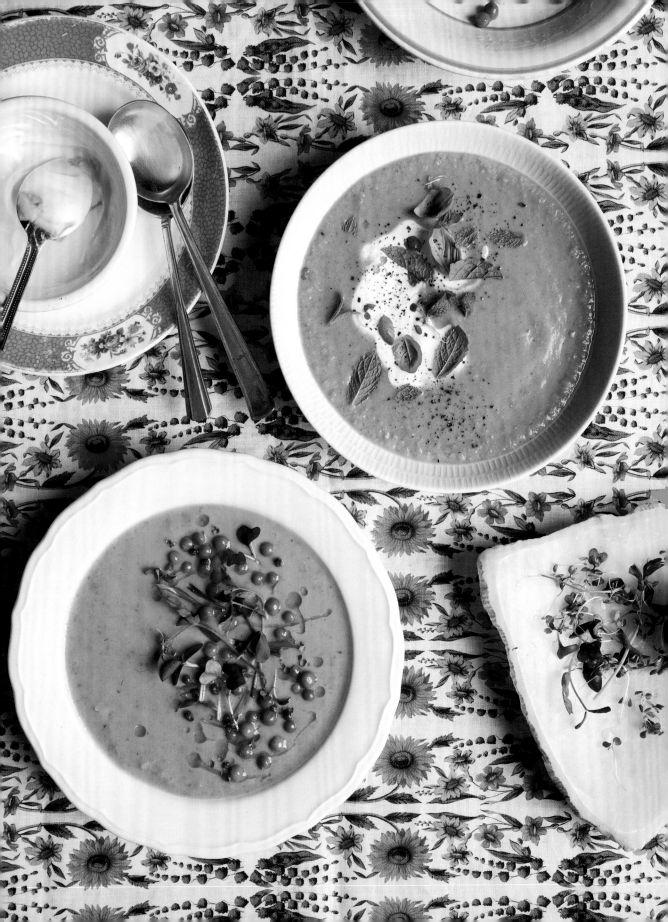

Super greens soup Serves 2

Ingredients

1 tablespoon extra virgin
olive oil, for frying

1 onion

4 garlic cloves, crushed

1 broccoli (try to use the stalk
as well), broken into florets
and chopped up

200g (7oz) frozen peas

200g (2 large handfuls of) spinach

600ml (2½ cups) vegetable or
chicken stock

freshly chopped herbs, such
as basil, mint, dill or coriander

juice of 1 lemon

salt and pepper

Toppings

yogurt or coconut milk

freshly chopped herbs, such
as basil, mint, dill or coriander

pumpkin seeds

Method

1. Heat some extra virgin olive oil in a large pan over a medium heat. Add the onion and sauté for around 8 minutes until soft and translucent. Add the garlic and cook for a further minute. Pop in the broccoli, peas and spinach, then pour over the stock. Season with salt and pepper and bring to the boil. Reduce the heat to a simmer, cover and cook for 25 minutes.

2. Stir through the herbs and lemon juice, then blitz the soup either with a stick blender or in a blender until completely smooth. Ladle into bowls and serve with a swirl of yogurt, and some more herbs and pumpkin seeds scattered on top.

15-minute pea, mint and butter bean soup Serves 4

Ingredients

2 tablespoons extra virgin olive oil

1 onion, diced

500ml (2 cups) vegetable stock
or broth

230g (8oz) cooked butter beans

500g (1lb 2oz) fresh shelled
peas or frozen peas

400ml (14fl oz) milk of your
choice (I used coconut milk)

about 20 mint leaves (4 sprigs),
or use basil, plus extra to serve

zest and juice of 1 lemon

salt and pepper

To serve

extra virgin olive oil, for drizzling

natural or plant-based yogurt

snipped chives

spring onions, thinly sliced

Method

1. Place a pan over a medium heat, add the extra virgin olive oil and gently fry the onion for 5 minutes until softened.

2. Add the stock or broth, butter beans, salt and pepper, then pop a lid on and let it come to a medium simmer.

3. Add the peas and milk and cook for a further few minutes, then turn off the heat and transfer to a blender along with the fresh mint leaves, lemon zest and juice and blitz until smooth, seasoning as you go.

4. Pour into bowls, drizzle with olive oil, garnish with more mint leaves and top with yogurt, chives and spring onions.

Green goddess salad Serves 2

Ingredients

½ small white cabbage,
finely diced

1 medium cucumber, finely diced

1 bunch of spring onions, sliced

4 tablespoons chives,
finely sliced

240g (8½oz) cooked white
beans, such as cannellini
or butter beans

2–4 brown tortillas

Dressing

juice of 2 lemons

60ml (¼ cup) extra virgin olive oil

2 tablespoons rice vinegar

2 garlic cloves

1 small shallot

20g (1 cup) fresh basil

30g (1 cup) fresh spinach

20g (⅓ cup) nutritional yeast

25g (¼ cup) walnuts

½ avocado

1 teaspoon salt

Method

1. Place all the vegetables and beans in a large bowl.

2. Grab yourself a blender cup and add all the dressing ingredients. Blend until smooth.

3. Add the dressing to the bowl with the diced vegetables and mix well.

4. Toast the tortillas and cut into triangles to eat with the salad.

The best gazpacho Serves 2–4

Ingredients

1.2kg (2lb 10oz) tomatoes (I use a
50/50 mix of plum tomatoes and
cherry tomatoes; use the best
quality ones you can)

1 cucumber, roughly chopped

2 garlic cloves, crushed

2 tablespoons chopped
white onion

275ml (9½fl oz) extra virgin
olive oil

2 teaspoons caster sugar

4 tablespoons red wine vinegar

1 teaspoon freshly chopped
red chilli

2 teaspoons sea salt

2 teaspoons black pepper

Dressing

¼ cucumber, cubed

extra virgin olive oil, for drizzling

1 slice of rye bread, halved
then quartered into triangles

Method

1. Place all the ingredients in a blender or food processor and process until smooth. You may need to do this in batches, depending on the size of your food processor. Transfer the gazpacho to a bowl, cover and chill for at least 1 hour.

2. Serve with cucumber, a drizzle of extra virgin olive oil and toasted rye bread on the side.

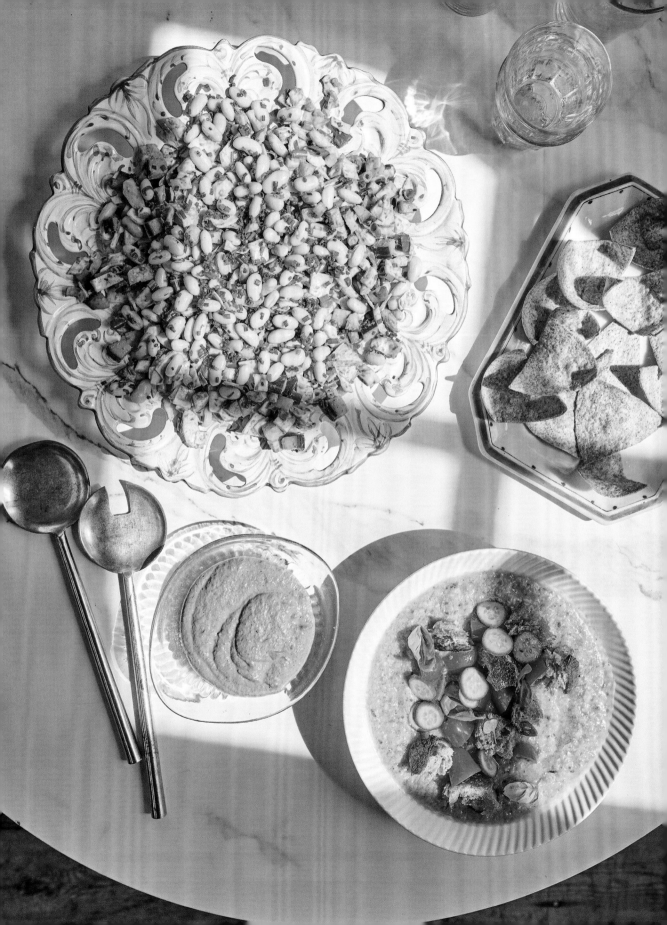

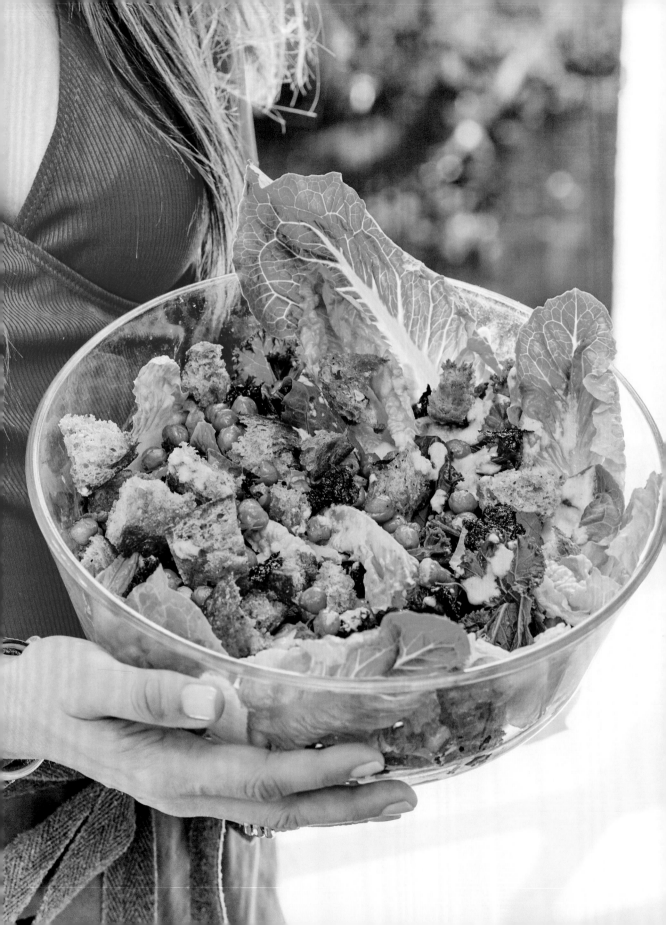

Kale Caesar salad Serves 2

Ingredients

100g (2 cups) of wholegrain or sourdough bread, torn into 2.5cm (1in) pieces

60ml (¼ cup) extra virgin olive oil, plus extra for drizzling

400g (14oz) can chickpeas, drained and rinsed

1 large bunch of kale, stems removed and roughly chopped into bite-sized pieces

1 large head of romaine lettuce, roughly chopped into bite-sized pieces

Dressing

140g (1 cup) whole (unroasted and unsalted) cashews

15g (¼ cup) nutritional yeast, plus extra to serve

60ml (¼ cup) fresh lemon juice (from 1–2 lemons)

3 garlic cloves

1 teaspoon Dijon mustard

1 teaspoon miso paste

175ml (¾ cup) filtered water

1 small sheet of roasted seaweed, crumbled (optional)

salt and pepper

Method

1. Preheat the oven to 180°C/160°C fan/350°F/gas mark 4. Toss the bread in extra virgin olive oil, salt and pepper to taste, then place on a lined baking tray. Toss the chickpeas in 2 tablespoons of extra virgin oil and season with some salt and pepper. Place both in the oven and cook until the chickpeas and bread are browned and crisp. Cook the bread for about 10 minutes and the chickpeas for about 20 minutes, moving both around halfway through cooking.

2. Next, make the dressing. Grab yourself a blender cup and add all the dressing ingredients. Blend until completely smooth, scraping down the sides and then set aside.

3. In a large bowl, add the kale and the dressing. Using your hands, massage the kale until slightly softened. Then add the lettuce, croutons and half the roasted chickpeas. Sprinkle with extra nutritional yeast and top with the remaining roasted chickpeas. Now you're ready to serve.

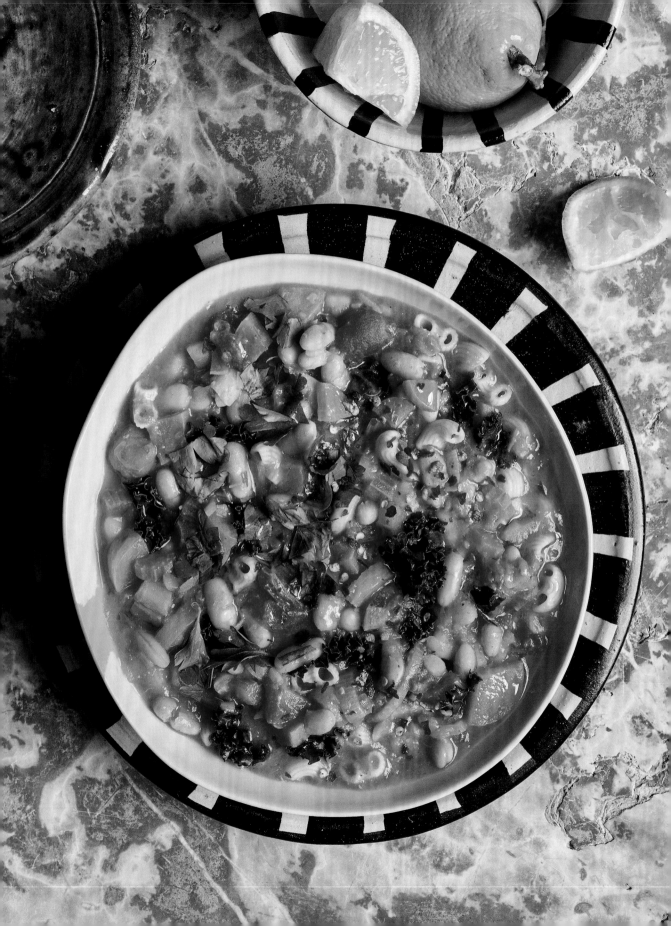

Pasta with beans Serves 6

Ingredients

extra virgin olive oil, for frying

1 medium onion, diced

2 carrots, washed and diced with skin on

2 celery sticks, diced

4 garlic cloves, crushed

400g (14oz) can plum tomatoes

950ml (4 cups) vegetable broth

700ml (3 cups) filtered water

2 bay leaves

1 teaspoon dried oregano

¼ teaspoon chilli flakes

2 x 400g (14oz) cans cannellini beans or chickpeas, rinsed and drained

120g (4¼oz) any kind of pasta, ideally smaller pasta is better (I use brown rice macaroni)

130g (2 cups) kale, chard or collard greens, destemmed and chopped or torn into bite-sized pieces

7g (¼ cup) flat-leaf parsley, finely chopped

1 tablespoon fresh lemon juice (about ½ medium lemon)

Toppings

fresh lemon juice

freshly chopped parsley

salt and pepper

Method

1. Place a large pan over a medium heat and add some extra virgin olive oil. Add the onion, carrots and celery and season with salt and pepper. Cook for 6–10 minutes, stirring often, until the vegetables have softened and the onion is translucent.

2. Add the garlic and cook for about 30 seconds until fragrant. Then add the tomatoes, pushing them against the side of the pan to break them apart. Cook the tomatoes until bubbling.

3. Add the vegetable broth, filtered water, bay leaves, oregano and chilli flakes and bring the mixture to a simmer. Cook for 10 minutes, stirring occasionally.

4. Use a heat-safe measuring cup to transfer about 350ml (1½ cups) of the soup (avoiding the bay leaves) to a blender. Add about 125g (¾ cup) of the drained beans and blend until smooth. Pour the blended mixture back into the soup.

5. Add the remaining beans, pasta, kale and parsley to the simmering soup. Continue cooking, stirring often to prevent the pasta from sticking to the bottom of the pan, for 15–20 minutes, or until the pasta and greens are pleasantly tender.

6. Remove the pan from the heat, then remove and discard the bay leaves. Stir in the lemon juice and season.

7. Add any toppings of your choice to serve. This soup is also great the next day or frozen, so if you have extra, try saving it for another day.

Chickpea Niçoise Serves 2

Ingredients

4 organic free-range eggs

extra virgin olive oil, for frying

400g (14oz) can chickpeas, drained and rinsed

200g (7oz) green beans, steamed

1 small handful of pitted green olives, halved

2 tablespoons capers

8 anchovies, diced

1 handful of radishes, sliced

1 handful of flat-leaf parsley, diced

1 handful of chives, diced

2 large handfuls of salad leaves

120g (4¼oz) cooked green lentils

Dressing

½ teaspoon herbs de Provence

1 teaspoon honey

2 tablespoons raw apple cider vinegar

2 tablespoons extra virgin olive oil

juice of 1 lemon

salt and pepper

Method

1. Cook the eggs for 7 minutes in strongly simmering water, then remove from the water and place under cold water. When cool enough to handle, peel and cut in half.

2. Place a frying pan over a medium heat and add some extra virgin olive oil. Add the chickpeas with some salt and pepper to taste. Fry over a medium heat for about 6 minutes until crispy, stirring constantly, then set aside.

3. Steam the green beans for about 4–5 minutes until tender (but still with some bite to them).

4. While the beans are steaming, make the dressing by placing all the dressing ingredients in a bowl and whisking together.

5. Assemble the salad by adding all the ingredients, except the eggs, to a large bowl and drizzling the dressing over the top, making sure everything is evenly coated with the dressing. Top with the eggs and serve.

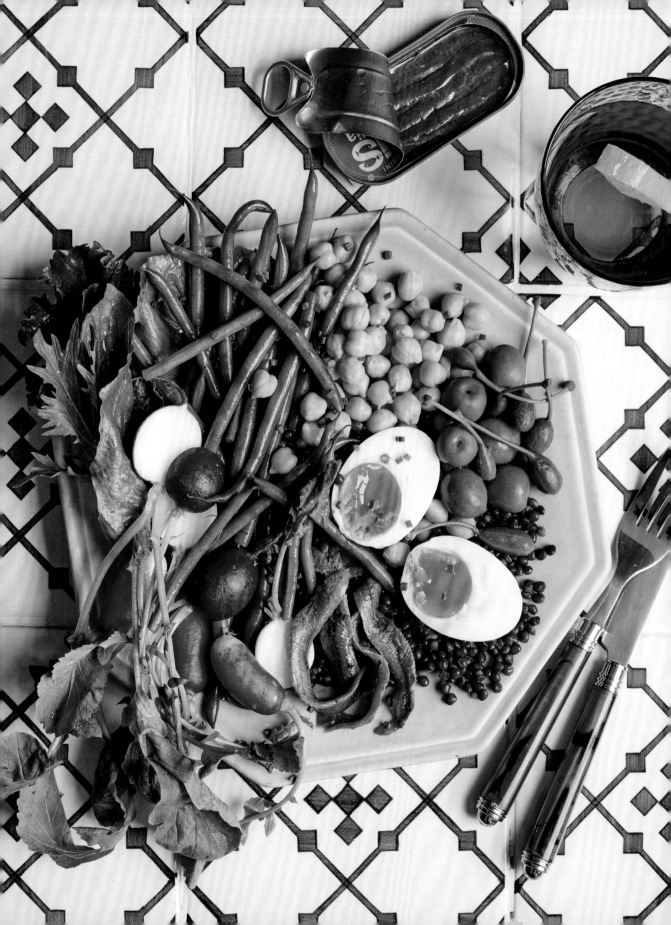

Swedish dill salad Serves 1–2

Ingredients

2 large handfuls of mixed greens

400g (14oz) can of chickpeas, drained and rinsed

½ cucumber, diced

about 8 cornichons or mini pickles, sliced

2 radishes, thinly sliced and cut into semicircles

1 handful of marinated artichokes

1 avocado, cut into bite-sized pieces

Dressing

2 tablespoons extra virgin olive oil

2 teaspoons honey

juice of 1 large lemon

1 tablespoon Dijon mustard

salt and pepper

Toppings

1 palm-sized serving of toasted pumpkin seeds

1 small handful of feta, crumbled

1 small handful of dill, torn into small pieces

Method

1. To make the dressing, mix all the ingredients together in a bowl.

2. Grab a large bowl and add the salad leaves and chickpeas. Pour over the dressing and mix to make sure everything is well coated.

3. Next, place the rest of the salad ingredients on top, then scatter over the toppings. Mix it all up when you're ready to eat.

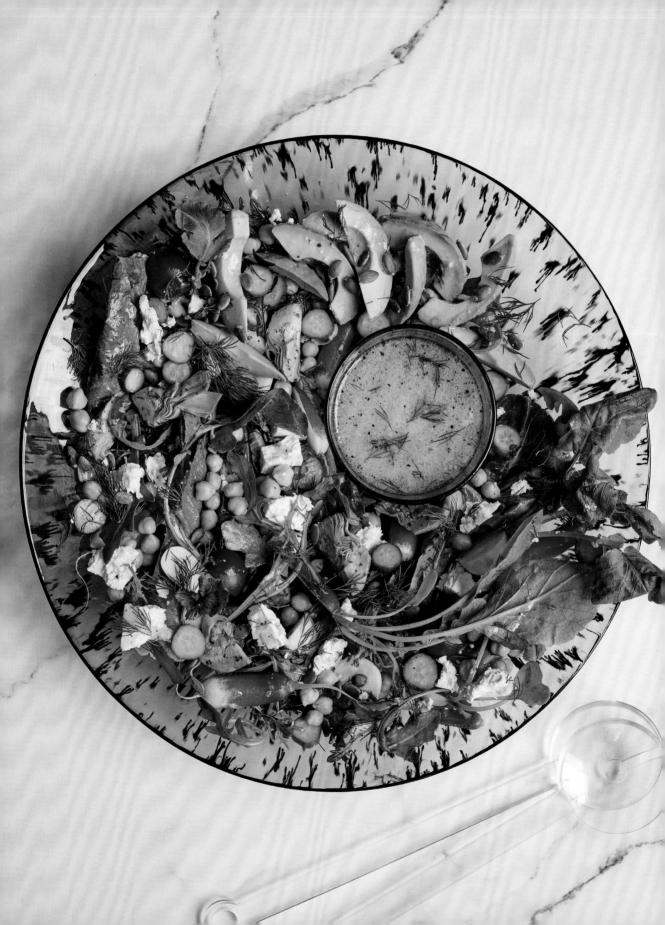

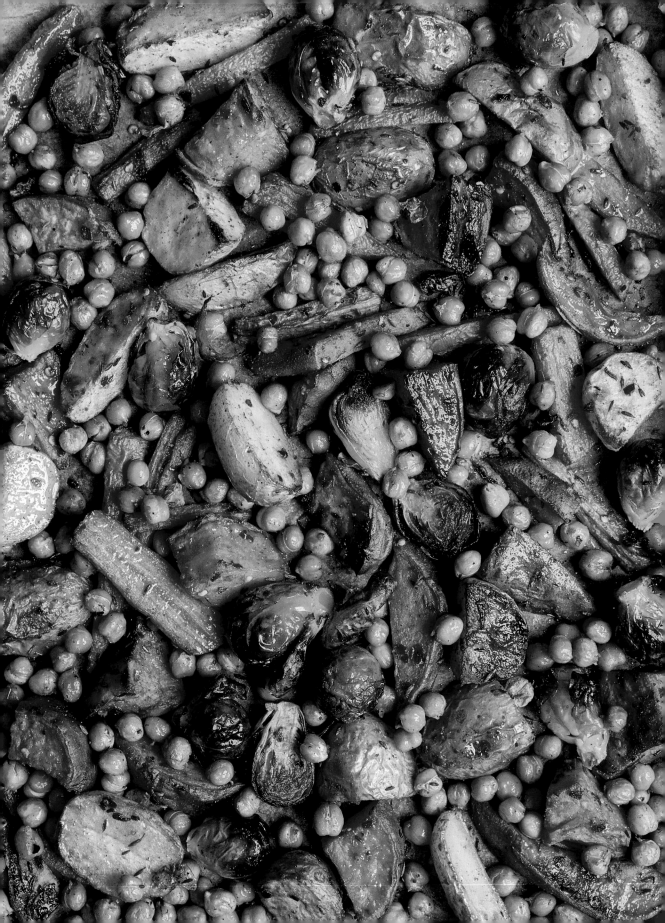

One-tray salad Serves 2

Ingredients

1 medium–large sweet potato, skin on and cut into 2cm (½in) cubes

1 medium-large potato, skin on and cut into 2cm (½in) cubes

4 carrots, cut into batons

90g (1 cup) Brussels sprouts, halved, or courgette, in semi-circles

1 teaspoon chilli flakes

1 teaspoon ground cumin

2 tablespoons extra virgin olive oil

1 teaspoon maple syrup

400g (14oz) can chickpeas, rinsed and drained

1 teaspoon cumin seeds

2 large handfuls of rocket

salt and pepper

Dressing

60ml (¼ cup) extra virgin olive oil

4 tablespoons tahini

2–3 tablespoons lemon juice, to taste

2 teaspoons Dijon mustard

2 teaspoons maple syrup or honey

2 tablespoons cold water, plus more as needed

2 tablespoons pumpkin, sunflower and sesame seeds

Method

1. Preheat the oven to 180°C/160°C fan/350°F/ gas mark 4.

2. Toss the potatoes, carrots, Brussels sprouts or courgette with the chilli flakes, ground cumin, extra virgin olive oil, maple syrup and some salt and pepper. Spread the vegetables out on a lined baking tray and cook for 45 minutes until just starting to brown, turning halfway through cooking.

3. In a small bowl, mix together all the dressing ingredients, except the seeds.

4. Once the vegetables have been cooking for 45 minutes, remove from the oven and mix through the chickpeas and cumin seeds. Return to the oven and cook for a further 15 minutes.

5. When the vegetables and chickpeas are cooked, transfer them to a bowl to cool, then add the rocket and pour over the dressing, making sure everything is evenly coated. Top with the seeds to serve.

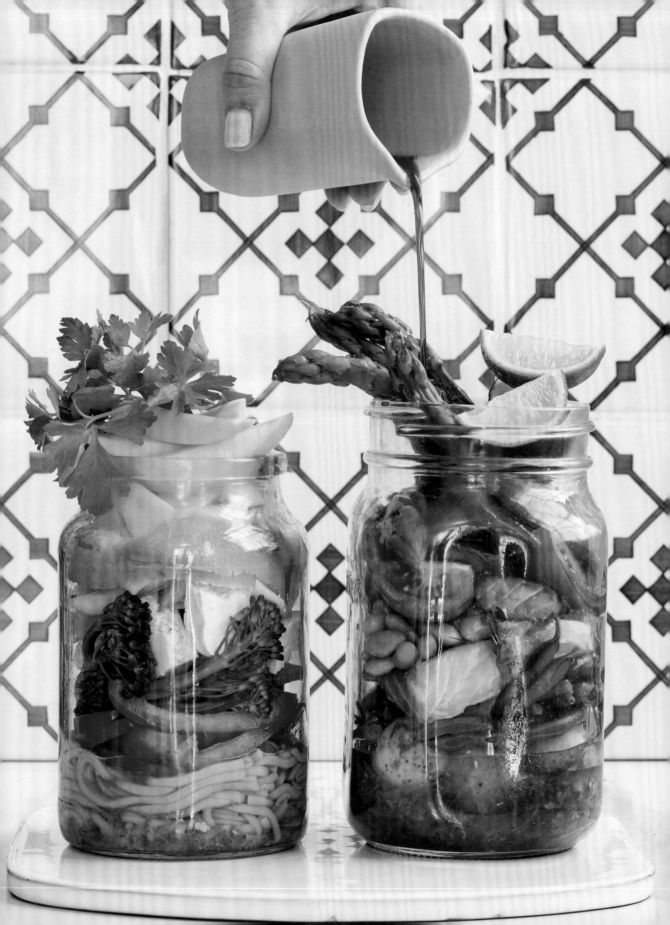

Noodle salad jars Serves 1

Lots of you always ask me for lunch ideas, so here are my noodle jars, which are quick, healthy and tasty. These can be tailored to any taste by following a mix and match formula, and leftovers are perfect for this.

Dressing

1 tablespoon freshly grated ginger

juice of 1 lime

1 tablespoon extra virgin olive oil

1 tablespoon light soy sauce or tamari

1 teaspoon honey

1 tablespoon Japanese rice vinegar

1 teaspoon fish sauce

1 red chilli, diced

Method

1. Mix together all of the dressing ingredients.

2. The basic formula to pop in your jar is:

1 carbohydrate:
rice, noodles, pasta, boiled potatoes, roasted sweet potato, butternut squash, quinoa, couscous.

1 protein:
chicken, prawns, smoked fish, tuna, steak, ham, tofu, chickpeas, eggs, cheese, lentils, nuts, seeds.

4–5 vegetables/fruit:
peppers, tomatoes, grated carrot, spinach, mango, papaya, avocado, radishes, cucumber, apple, pears, roasted vegetables (such as aubergine, fennel, peppers).

TikTok tortilla Each makes 1

Avocado, sweetcorn, jalapeño and cheese

1 wholegrain wrap

½ avocado, sliced

1 handful of tomatoes, sliced

1 small handful of rocket

85g (½ cup) sweetcorn

6 jalapeño slices

30g (1 small handful)
grated cheese

1. Lay your tortilla on a chopping board. Take a knife and make a cut from the middle of the tortilla down to the edge.

2. Imagine the tortilla being divided up into four quarters. Going clockwise, place a different ingredient into each quarter. Starting with the avocado in the bottom left quarter, the tomatoes and rocket in the second one, the sweetcorn and jalapeños in the third one and the cheese in the last one.

3. Fold the wrap up, starting from the bottom left quarter, folding it up and over the top left, then folding it over to the top right, then folding it down to the bottom right.

4. Enjoy as is or grill in a panini press or pan.

Grilled mushrooms, pesto, hummus and avocado

extra virgin olive oil, for frying

1 large portobello or field
mushroom, sliced

1 wholegrain wrap

½ avocado, sliced

2 tablespoons hummus

1 tablespoon any kind of pesto
you like (I used basil pesto)

1 small handful of rocket

1. Pop your mushroom on a baking tray, drizzle with extra virgin olive oil and roast at 180°C/160°C fan/350°F/gas mark 4 for about 8 minutes until cooked through. Set to one side to cool and slice into strips.

2. Lay your tortilla on a chopping board. Take a knife and make a cut from the middle of the tortilla down to the edge.

3. Imagine the tortilla being divided up into four quarters. Going clockwise, place a different ingredient into each quarter. Starting with the avocado in the bottom left quarter, the hummus in the second one, the mushroom in the third one and the pesto and rocket in the last one.

4. Fold the wrap up, starting from the bottom left quarter, folding it up and over the top left, then folding it over to the top right, then folding it down to the bottom right.

5. Place a pan over a medium heat, then place the wrap in it and cook for about 2 minutes on each side until toasted.

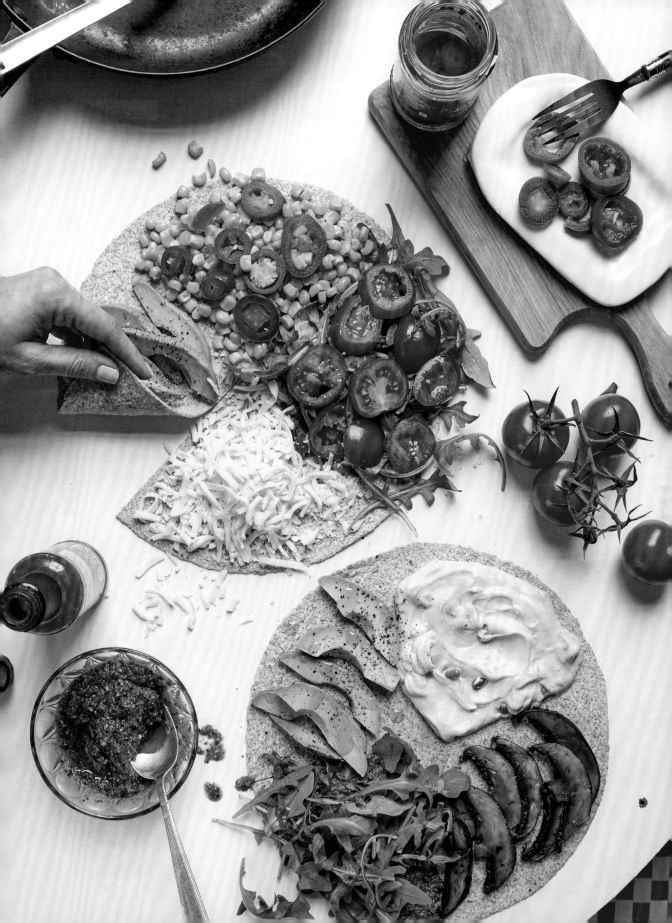

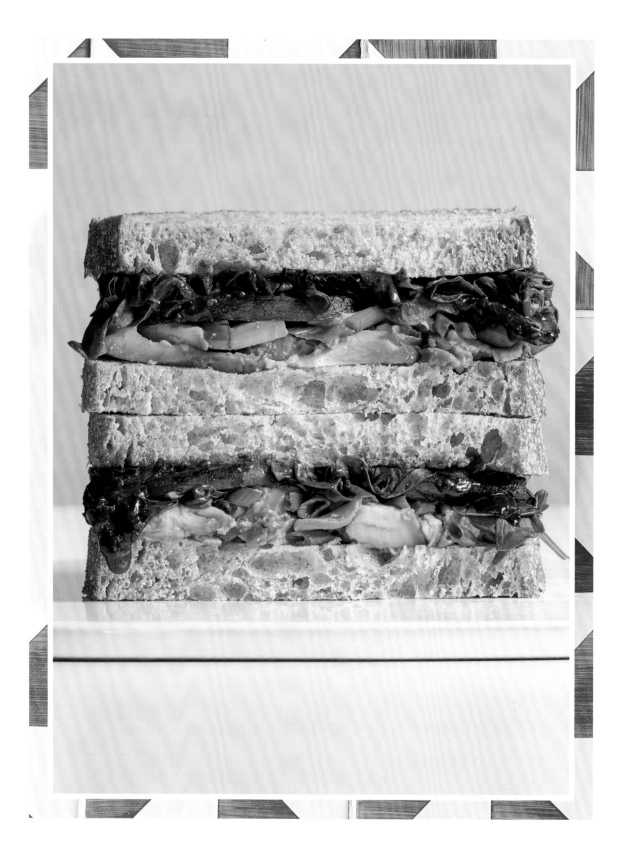

Miso mushroom, avocado and spinach sandwich Makes 1

Ingredients

extra virgin olive oil

100g (3½oz) portobello mushrooms, sliced

1 handful of fresh spinach

2 garlic cloves, crushed

1 tablespoon brown rice miso paste

1 tablespoon maple syrup

1 teaspoon tamari

1 teaspoon brown rice vinegar

juice of 1 lime

½ avocado, mashed

1 spring onion, sliced

2 thick slices of sourdough bread

salt and pepper

Method

1. Heat the extra virgin olive oil in a pan over a medium–high heat. Add the mushrooms, spinach and garlic, and season with salt and pepper.

2. Mix through the miso paste, maple syrup, tamari, brown rice vinegar and lime juice and cook for about 5 minutes until the sauce has begun to thicken.

3. Mix the avocado and spring onion together in a bowl.

4. Lightly toast the bread on either side and then pop the mashed avocado on top of one slice and the mushroom mixture on top of that, and top with the remaining slice of bread. Now you're ready to serve. Enjoy!

Avocado vegetable toasted sandwich Makes 1

Ingredients

extra virgin olive oil, for frying

¼ shallot, diced (onion or garlic would work too)

60g (2¼oz) portobello mushrooms (or any kind of mushrooms you like), sliced

50g (¼ cup) cherry tomatoes, halved

15g (½ cup) spinach or kale, chopped and stems removed

½ avocado

2 thick slices of sourdough bread

30g (1oz) mozzarella or vegan meltable cheese, grated or sliced (optional)

salt and pepper

Method

1. Heat the extra virgin olive oil in a pan over a medium–high heat. Add the shallot and sauté until translucent. Add the mushrooms and sauté until lightly browned. Add the tomatoes and spinach or kale and sauté until wilted and warmed through. Remove from the heat and season with salt and pepper.

2. Mash the avocado in a bowl with a fork. Spread some avocado on the surface of one slice of bread. Top with the vegetables.

3. Add the cheese on top of the vegetables, cover with the remaining slice of bread, and ideally place on a preheated panini press, or in a hot griddle pan. When the bread is browned on the outside and the cheese has started to melt, remove from the heat and serve. Enjoy!

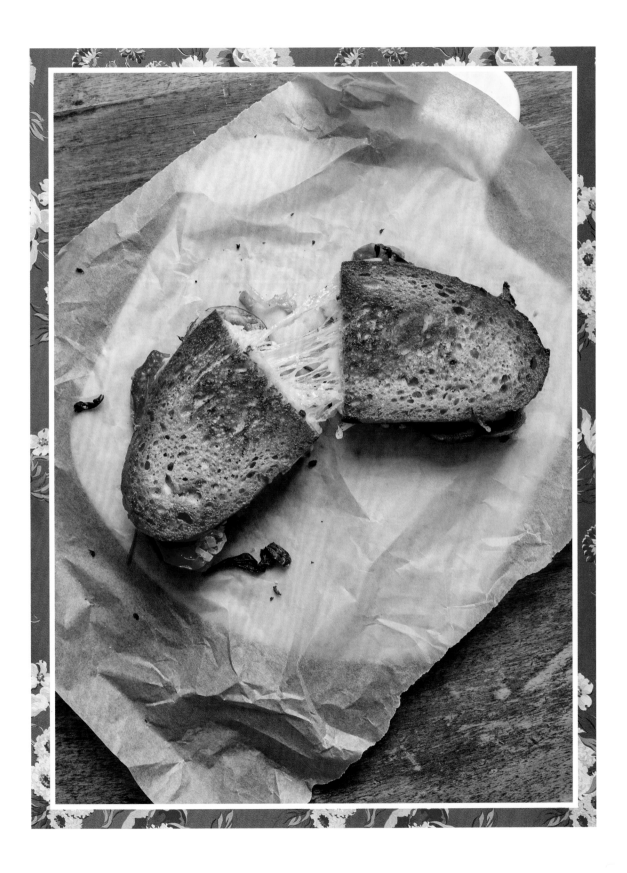

Mains

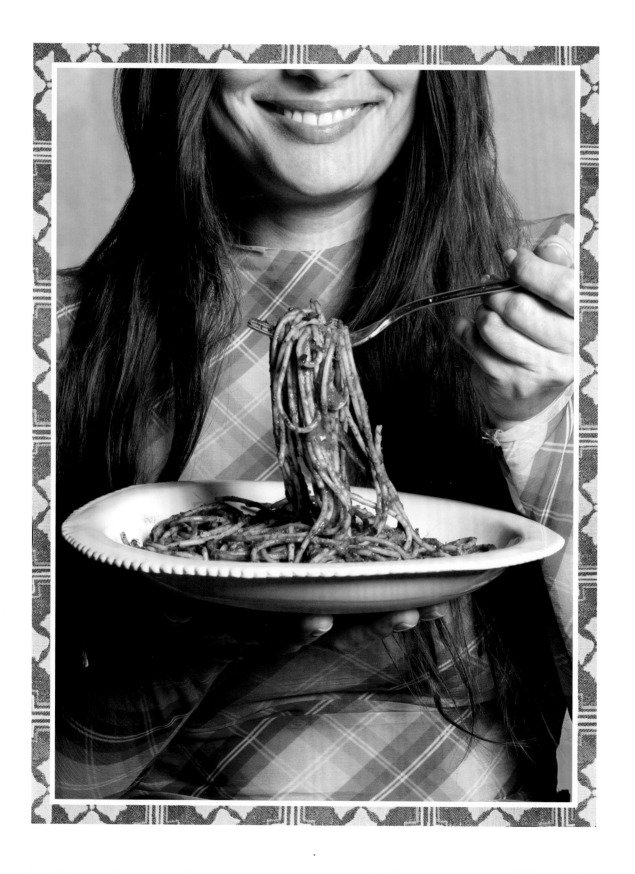

Super green pasta Serves 1

Ingredients

100g (3½oz) any kind of pasta (I use brown rice spaghetti)

2 garlic cloves, left whole

100g (3½oz) cavolo nero or kale, roughly chopped

60g (2¼oz) spinach

1 tablespoon extra virgin olive oil, plus extra to serve

juice of ½ lemon

30g (1oz) Parmesan or vegan cheese, grated, plus extra to serve

2 tablespoons nutritional yeast (optional)

salt and pepper

chilli flakes, to serve

Method

1. Cook the pasta in boiling water according to the packet instructions.

2. About 3–4 minutes before the pasta is ready, add the garlic, cavolo nero and spinach to the pasta water and cook until soft.

3. Using tongs, carefully remove all the veg and transfer to a blender, along with the extra virgin olive oil, lemon juice, cheese, nutritional yeast, salt and pepper. Blend until super-smooth and creamy.

4. Drain the pasta, reserving a few tablespoons of the pasta water.

5. Return the pasta to the saucepan with the green sauce from the blender, loosening with a splash of the reserved pasta cooking water.

6. To serve, top with more cheese, extra virgin olive oil and chilli flakes and enjoy!

Roasted aubergine and tomato pasta Serves 2

Ingredients

2 medium aubergines

extra virgin olive oil,
for drizzling

1 small onion, finely diced

4 garlic cloves, crushed

400g (14oz) can plum tomatoes

½ tablespoon mixed
dried herbs

½ teaspoon chilli flakes,
to taste (optional)

½ teaspoon dried oregano

200g (7oz) pasta
(I use brown rice pasta)

5g (¼ cup) freshly chopped
basil, plus extra to serve

40g (1½oz) Parmesan or
vegan cheese, grated, plus
extra to serve

salt and pepper

Method

1. Preheat the oven on to 180°C/160°C fan/350°F/gas mark 4.

2. Use a vegetable peeler to shave off long alternating strips of aubergine peel. The aubergine will look striped like a zebra when you're done. Then slice the aubergine into 1cm (½in) thick circles, discarding the end pieces. Place the aubergine on a lined baking tray, brush generously with extra virgin olive oil on both sides, and season with salt and pepper. Roast for 35–45 minutes until golden brown and tender, turning after 20 minutes. Set aside.

3. Meanwhile, make the tomato sauce by placing a pan over a medium heat and adding some extra virgin olive oil. Cook the onion until translucent, then add the garlic and cook for about 30 seconds. Pour in the canned plum tomatoes (push the tomatoes against the side of the pan to break them down), dried herbs, chilli flakes and oregano and season with salt and pepper. Bring to a simmer and cook for around 20 minutes, then set aside.

4. Bring a pan of water to the boil and cook the pasta according to the packet instructions until al dente. Reserve about half a cup of the pasta cooking water before draining.

5. When the aubergines are cooked, gently stir them into the sauce. Add 1 teaspoon of extra virgin olive oil and the basil, then cook over a low–medium heat for 2–3 minutes until everything is well combined.

6. Add the pasta to the sauce with a couple of tablespoons of the reserved pasta cooking water, and gently stir. Add about two thirds of the cheese, reserving the rest to serve. Season to taste. You may need to add a bit more of the reserved pasta cooking water to loosen up the sauce, if desired.

7. To serve, divide the pasta between two bowls and top with the remaining cheese, fresh basil and drizzle with extra virgin olive oil. Enjoy!

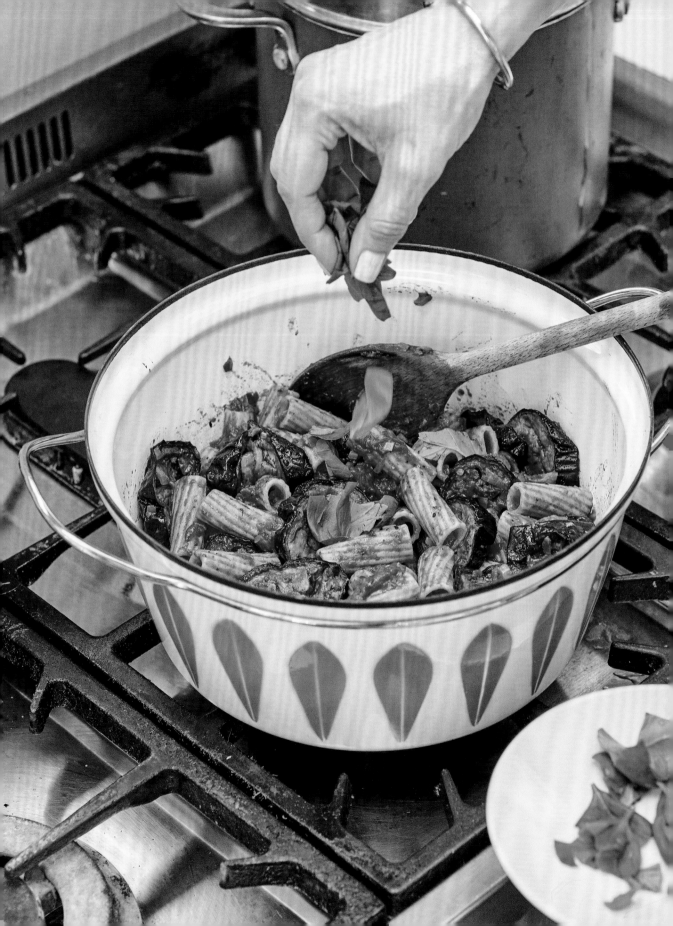

Soba noodles and crispy kale Serves 2

Ingredients

200g (7oz) firm tofu, chopped into bite-sized cubes and dabbed dry with kitchen paper

4 tablespoons extra virgin olive oil

2 tablespoons sesame oil

2 large handfuls of kale, stalks removed and torn into bite-sized pieces

20g (1/3 cup) nutritional yeast

240g (8½oz) soba noodles (I use buckwheat soba noodles)

200g (7oz) any kind of mushrooms, sliced

½ cucumber, sliced into ribbons

Sauce

120g (½ cup) light tahini

2 tablespoons light soy sauce or tamari

2 teaspoons sesame oil

1 tablespoon honey

½ teaspoon chilli flakes

zest and juice of 1 lime

60ml (¼ cup) extra virgin olive oil

Method

1. Pop the tofu into a bowl with 2 tablespoons of the extra virgin olive oil and sesame oil and leave to marinate for 1 hour.

2. When you're ready to start cooking, preheat the oven to 190°C/170°C fan/375°F/gas mark 5.

3. Next, cover the kale with the remaining 2 tablespoons of extra virgin olive oil and the nutritional yeast, making sure it is evenly coated – you may need to use your hands. Then lay the kale out across two large, lined baking trays – you want to make sure the kale is evenly spaced and not overlapping. Pop in the oven to cook for 15–20 minutes until the kale is crispy.

4. Meanwhile, make your sauce by adding all the ingredients to a bowl and mixing together well.

5. Place a large frying pan over a medium heat, add the tofu and cook until it is golden brown. Transfer to a plate and set aside. Use the same pan to sauté your mushrooms until they are cooked through and tender.

6. Meanwhile, cook your soba noodles according to the packet instructions, then rinse well under cold water

7. Grab a large serving plate and add the soba noodles and mushrooms, then pour over the sauce, making sure the noodles are evenly coated. Top with the kale, tofu and cucumber, then mix it all together.

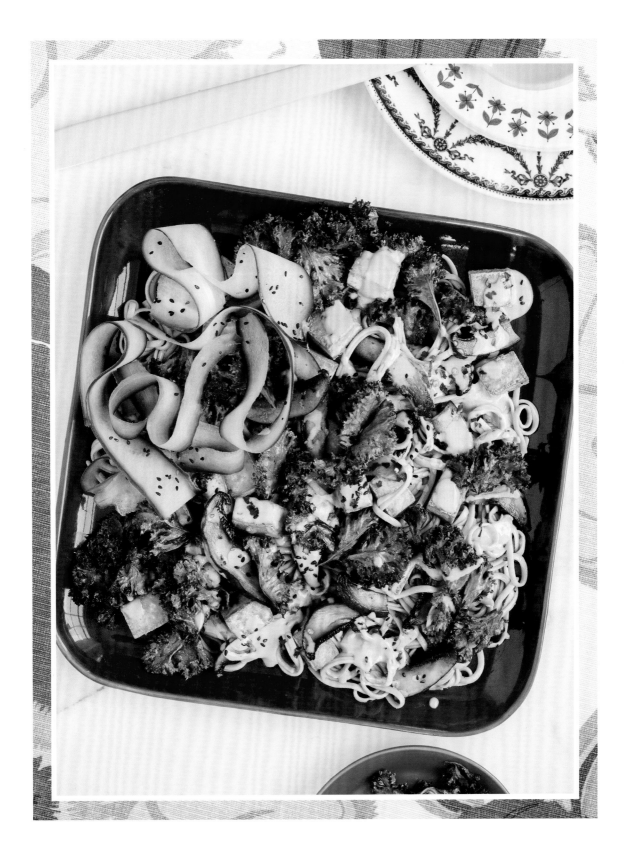

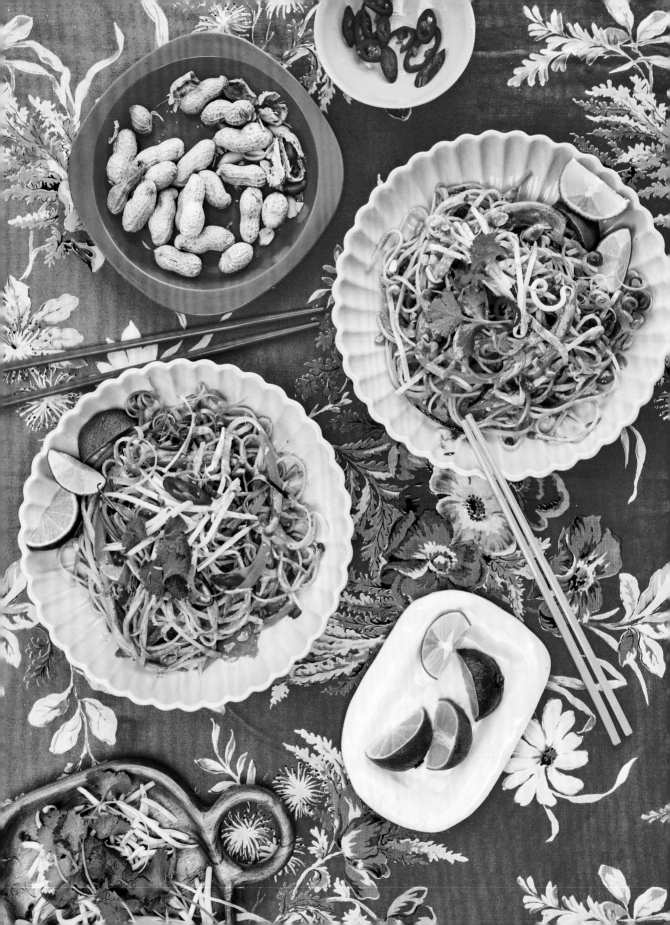

Veggie pad Thai noodles Serves 2

Ingredients

120g (4¼oz) flat rice noodles

extra virgin olive oil, for frying

2 medium carrots, scrubbed and cut into thin batons

1 courgette, cut into thin batons

1 yellow pepper, cut into thin batons

1 large handful of beansprouts

1 handful of fresh coriander, diced

1 red chilli, diced

2 spring onions, sliced

50g (1¾oz) roasted peanuts, crumbled

Dressing

3 tablespoons smooth peanut butter

1 tablespoon fish sauce

1 tablespoon light soy sauce or tamari

juice of 1 lime, plus extra to serve (optional)

thumb-sized piece of fresh ginger, skin on and grated

1 tablespoon maple syrup

Method

1. Cook the noodles in simmering water according to the packet instructions, then run under cold water and set aside.

2. To make the dressing, pop all the ingredinets in a small bowl and mix well.

3. Place a pan over over a medium-high heat and add some extra virgin olive oil. Add the carrots, courgette, yellow pepper and beansprouts and stir-fry for 2–3 minutes or until tender and crisp. Be careful not to overcook the vegetables – they'll get soggy and heavy.

4. Once the vegetables are cooked, add the noodles and dressing, then stir in until they are warmed through, making sure everything is evenly coated.

5. To serve, divide into bowls and top with the coriander, chilli, spring onions, peanuts and more fresh lime juice if you like.

Miso, ginger, carrot and brown rice stir-fry Serves 2

Ingredients

120g (4½oz) brown rice

extra virgin olive oil, for frying

2 garlic cloves, minced

1 small head of broccoli, chopped and broken into bite-sized florets (don't forget to slice the stalk into bite-sized pieces too)

2 medium carrots, skin on and cut into ribbons or semicircles

1 red pepper, diced into bite-sized pieces

Dressing

3 tablespoons brown rice miso paste

2 teaspoons maple syrup

2 tablespoons extra virgin olive oil

juice of 2 limes

1 tablespoon grated fresh ginger

1 teaspoon brown rice vinegar

Toppings

fresh coriander, chopped

fresh chilli, diced or chilli flakes

fresh lime juice

2 spring onions, sliced

1 tablespoon sesame seeds

Method

1. Cook the rice according to the packet instructions, making sure to rinse it with cold water first. Once cooked, set aside.

2. Meanwhile, make the dressing by mixing all the ingredients together in a small bowl.

3. Next, place a wok or large frying pan over a medium–high heat and add some extra virgin olive oil. Add the garlic, broccoli, carrots and red pepper and cook for a few minutes so the vegetables are soft but still have bite.

4. Stir the rice through the vegetables and cover with the dressing, making sure everything is evenly coated.

5. Spoon into bowls and top with fresh coriander, chilli, lime juice, spring onions and sesame seeds.

Tip: Rinse the rice before cooking. Place in a pan, cover with cold water to 1cm (½in) above the top of the rice and cook according to the packet instructions. There should not be any water to drain off the rice.

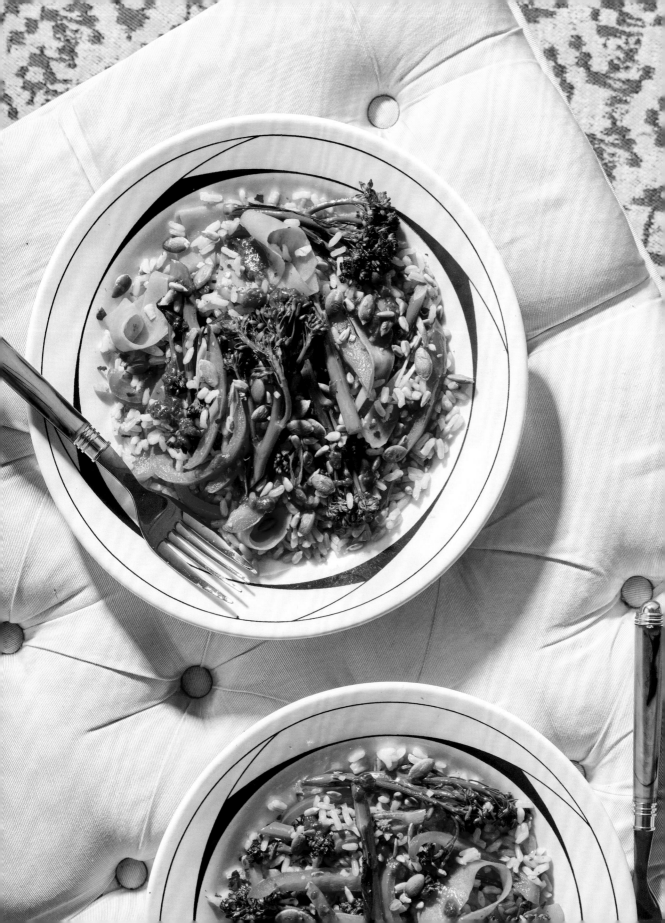

Vegetable tagine with almond and chickpea quinoa Serves 4–6

Ingredients

2 tablespoons extra virgin olive oil

1 red onion, sliced

1 medium aubergine, diced

2 large carrots, skin on and sliced into rounds

1 red pepper, diced

1 yellow pepper, diced

1 small butternut squash, peeled, deseeded and cut into bite-sized pieces

1 courgette, sliced into semicircles

6 garlic cloves, crushed

2 tablespoons tomato purée

2 teaspoons ground coriander

2 teaspoons ground cumin

1 teaspoon ground cinnamon

½ teaspoon ground turmeric

2 tablespoons harissa paste

1 tablespoon honey

400g (14oz) can plum tomatoes

400ml (14fl oz) vegetable stock

10 dried apricots, halved

1 small handful of fresh mint, finely chopped

salt and pepper

Almond and chickpea quinoa

300g (10½oz) quinoa

extra virgin olive oil, for drizzling

400g (14oz) can chickpeas, rinsed and drained

480ml (2 cups) hot vegetable stock

2 tablespoons harissa paste

juice of 1 lemon

1 large handful of toasted flaked almonds

salt and pepper

Method

1. Heat the extra virgin olive oil in a large, wide pan with a lid over a medium-high heat and add the onion, aubergine, carrots, peppers, butternut squash and courgette. Cook for 10–15 minutes, stirring regularly, until the vegetables have started to soften and are lightly browned.

2. Add the garlic, tomato purée, ground coriander, cumin, cinnamon and turmeric and cook for a further 2 minutes, stirring constantly.

3. Add the harissa, honey, canned plum tomatoes, vegetable stock and apricots. Give everything a good stir, making sure to break apart the plum tomatoes as you do. Cover the pan and bring to the boil, then turn the heat down to low and simmer gently for 45 minutes–1 hour until all of the vegetables have softened.

4. Season to taste with salt and pepper and stir in the chopped mint.

5. Meanwhile, to make the almond and chickpea quinoa, rinse the quinoa, then cook in a large frying pan until dry. Add a small drizzle of extra virgin olive oil along with the chickpeas and fry until golden brown. Then add the vegetable stock and harissa and give it a stir. Cook the quinoa until all the stock has been absorbed.

6. Add lemon juice to taste, the toasted flaked almonds and salt and pepper. Serve alongside the vegetable tagine.

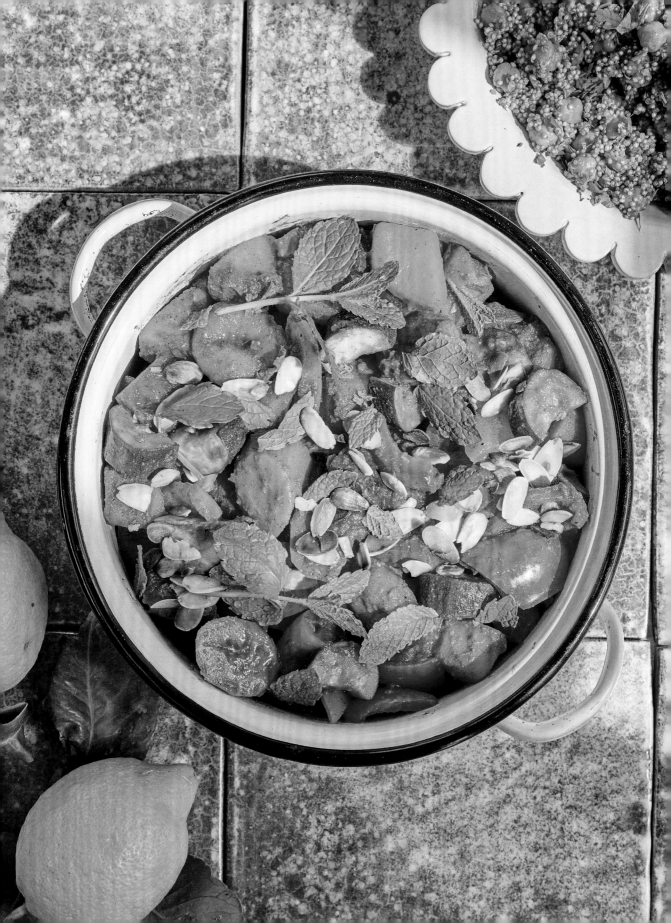

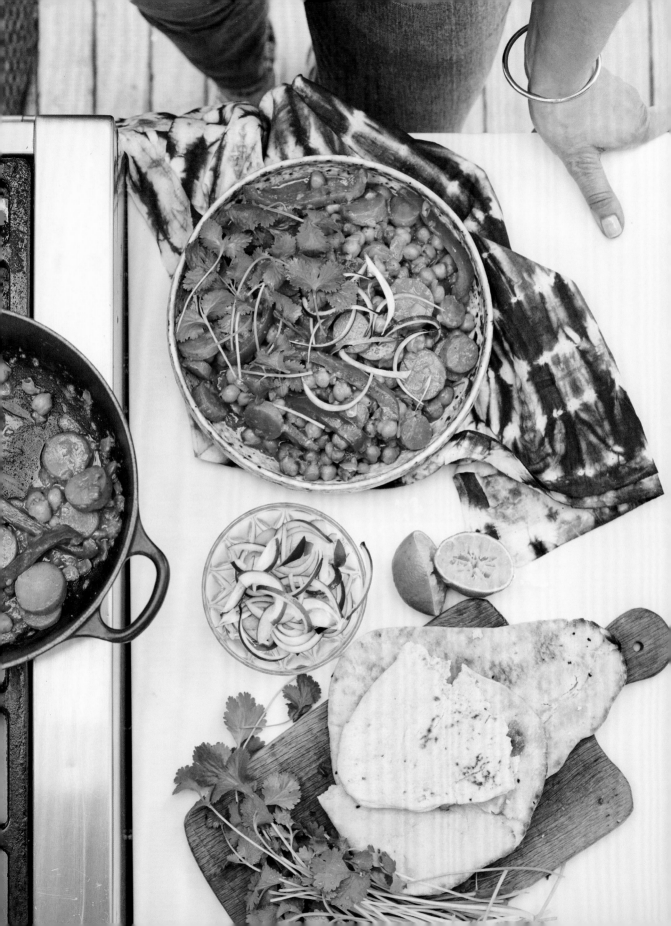

Spiced chickpea coconut curry Serves 2

Ingredients

extra virgin olive oil, for frying

1 onion, diced

2 tablespoons fresh
coriander, diced

4 garlic cloves, crushed

25g (1oz) fresh ginger,
skin on and grated

400g (14oz) can chickpeas,
rinsed and drained

2 medium carrots, skin on
and sliced into half-moons

1 red pepper, sliced

1 teaspoon ground turmeric

1 teaspoon ground cumin

½ teaspoon chilli flakes

1 teaspoon garam masala

400ml (14fl oz) can
coconut milk

salt and pepper

Toppings

fresh coriander

red onion, thinly sliced

juice of 1 lime

To serve

Serve with brown rice,
quinoa or naan

Method

1. Heat a pan over a medium–high heat and add some extra virgin olive oil. Add the onion and cook for 5–10 minutes until translucent and golden around the edges.

2. Add the coriander, garlic and ginger and cook for about 30 seconds until fragrant.

3. Next, add the chickpeas, carrots and red pepper, and cook for about 2 minutes, stirring occasionally.

4. Stir in the ground turmeric powder and cumin, chilli flakes and garam masala, and cook for 30–45 seconds.

5. Stir in the coconut milk, season with salt and pepper, then bring to a simmer and cook for 10 minutes, stirring occasionally.

6. Top with coriander, red onion and fresh lime juice. Serve with brown rice, quinoa or naan.

Walnut meat tacos Makes 6–8 tacos

Ingredients

1 head of cauliflower, florets,
core and leaves chopped
(use the whole cauliflower)

250g (9oz) walnuts

2 teaspoons lime juice

50g (1¾oz) sun-dried tomatoes

2 garlic cloves, crushed

½ teaspoon sea salt

½ tablespoon smoked paprika

½ tablespoon ground cumin

2 teaspoons medium
chilli powder

2 teaspoons nutritional
yeast (optional)

1½ tablespoons extra virgin
olive oil

60ml (¼ cup) water

To serve

wholegrain tortillas

avocado, thinly sliced

pinto beans, warmed through

cherry tomatoes, finely diced

fresh coriander, finely chopped

fresh lime juice

red onion, thinly sliced

hot sauce

Method

1. Preheat the oven to 180°C/160°C fan/350°F/
   gas mark 4.

2. Pulse the cauliflower, walnuts and lime juice in
   a food processor until they are roughly combined.
   Place in a bowl and set aside.

3. Add the sun-dried tomatoes, garlic, salt, smoked
   paprika, cumin, chilli powder and nutritional yeast
   (if using) to the empty food processor and blend.
   Slowly add 1 tablespoon of the extra virgin olive
   oil to thicken the mixture.

4. Stir the spiced mixture into the bowl of
   cauliflower and walnuts, using your hands if you
   need to, making sure everything is thoroughly
   combined. Add the water to keep the mixture
   from drying out.

5. Transfer to a lined baking tray and bake for
   20–25 minutes. Stir halfway through for an
   even bake.

6. Serve in wholegrain tortillas with avocado,
   pinto beans, chopped cherry tomatoes, coriander,
   lime juice, red onion and hot sauce, or whatever
   you fancy!

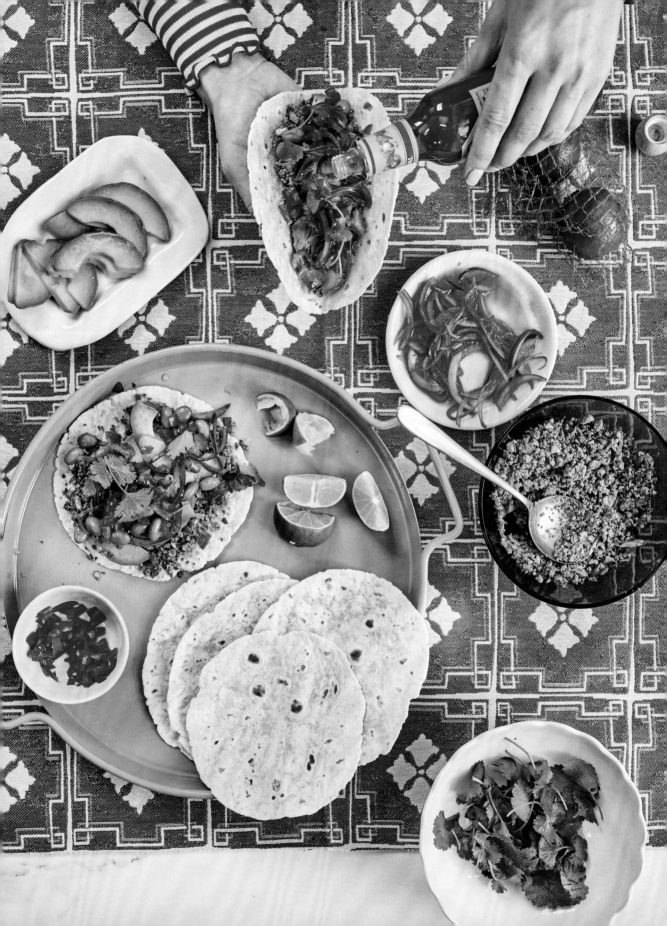

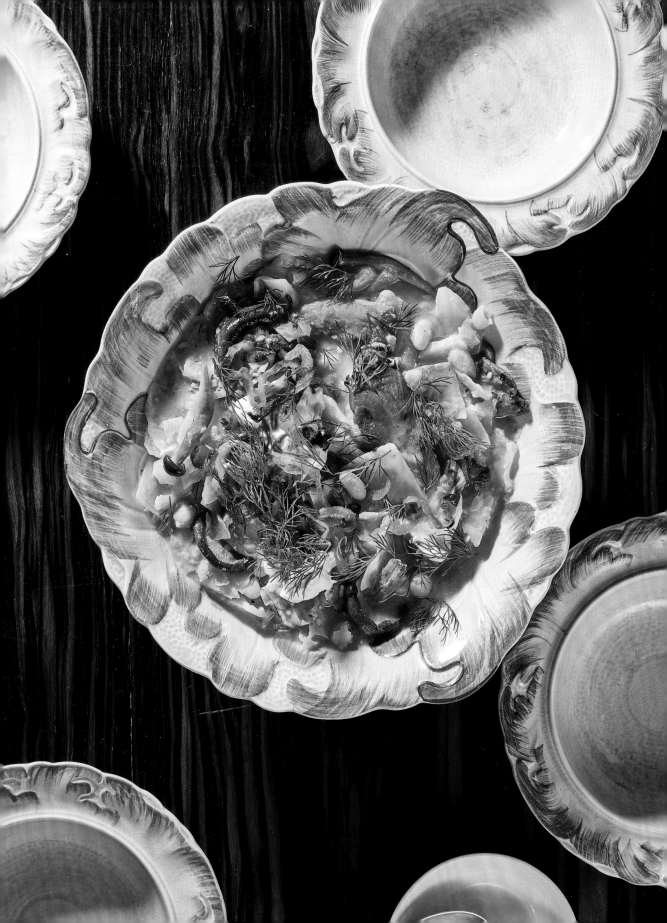

White bean stew with cabbage and onions Serves 2–4

Ingredients

4 tablespoons extra virgin
olive oil, plus extra to
serve (optional)

1 large onion, thinly sliced

2 x 400g (14oz) cans cannellini
beans (or any white beans,
such as haricot or butter
beans), drained and rinsed

950ml (4 cups) vegetable
or chicken broth (or 950ml
(4 cups) warm water plus
2 tablespoons bouillon)

200g (7oz) mushrooms,
sliced into bite-sized pieces
(I use a mixture based on
what's in season)

½ head of white cabbage,
coarsely chopped into
bite-sized pieces

2 tablespoons apple
cider vinegar

4.5g (½ cup) dill,
coarsely chopped

natural yogurt, about
2 tablespoons per person

salt and pepper

salt and pepper

Method

1. Heat the extra virgin olive oil in a medium pan over a medium–high heat. Add the onion and season with salt and pepper. Cook for 8–10 minutes, without stirring too much, until it is just turning brown. You don't want caramelized onion or burnt onion, but right in the middle, so adjust the heat and frequency of stirring as needed.

2. Using a slotted spoon, transfer half of the onion to a small bowl and set aside (this is for topping).

3. Add the beans to the pan and, using a wooden spoon, spatula or potato masher, crush about half of the beans into the pan. You want to have some of the beans crushed and some still whole.

4. Then add the broth and simmer for 15–20 minutes until you reach your desired consistency. Add the mushrooms, cabbage and vinegar and simmer, with a lid on, for about 15 minutes until the cabbage and mushrooms are tender, and all the flavours have come together. Season with salt, pepper and more vinegar if you like.

5. Remove from the heat and stir in half the dill. Divide between bowls and top with more dill, the reserved onions and more pepper. Drizzle with extra virgin olive oil and stir in some yogurt if you like.

Tomato and ricotta tart   Serves 6

Ingredients

110g (3¾oz) 100 per cent rolled oats

60g (2¼oz) gram flour

1 date, finely chopped

1 teaspoon dried oregano

1 teaspoon dried thyme

pinch of salt

70ml (2½fl oz) extra virgin olive oil, plus extra for greasing

5 tablespoons cold water

4 medium vine tomatoes, sliced

2 large handfuls of mixed colour cherry tomatoes, halved

Filling

extra virgin olive oil, for frying

2 medium onions, diced

5 garlic cloves, chopped

500g (1lb 2oz) ricotta

20g (¾oz) basil, finely chopped

½ teaspoon salt

½ teaspoon black pepper

3 free-range organic eggs, plus 2 yolks

To serve

serve with a big green salad

Method

1. Preheat the oven to 180°C/160°C fan/350°F/gas mark 4 and grease a 23cm (9in) springform tin with extra virgin olive oil.

2. Blend the oats into flour in a blender, then add the gram flour, date, oregano, thyme and salt. Pulse to combine, then gradually mix in the extra virgin olive oil. Add the water, a tablespoon at a time, until a dough forms.

3. Press the dough into the prepared tin, forming a flat base. Poke the base with a fork to allow air to escape and then bake for 10–12 minutes until cooked through and slightly browned.

4. Meanwhile, make the filling. Heat some extra virgin olive oil in a large frying pan over a low–medium heat and sauté the onions for 20 minutes or so, stirring from time to time until they are soft and sweet but haven't taken on any colour. Add the garlic for the last 2 minutes of cooking. Set aside to cool.

5. Grab a large bowl, add the ricotta and whisk it, ideally using an electric whisk. Then add the cooled onion and garlic mixture, the basil, salt and pepper, and mix until well incorporated.

6. In a separate large mixing bowl, whisk the eggs and yolks together, preferably with an electric whisk, until light and airy. Add the ricotta and onion mixture carefully and work just until it is well incorporated. Pour over the pastry and bake for 45–50 minutes, or until just set.

7. Arrange the tomatoes on a lined baking tray, cut side up, drizzle with extra virgin olive oil and season with salt and pepper, then sprinkle with the oregano and thyme. Roast in the oven for around 30 minutes until the edges are just starting to catch.

8. Once everything is cooked, arrange the roasted tomatoes, cut-side up, on top of the tart, so they are touching. Serve immediately, or pop the tart back in the oven for a few minutes to serve warm-ish. (It can also be left to cool and served cold.) Serve with a big green salad.

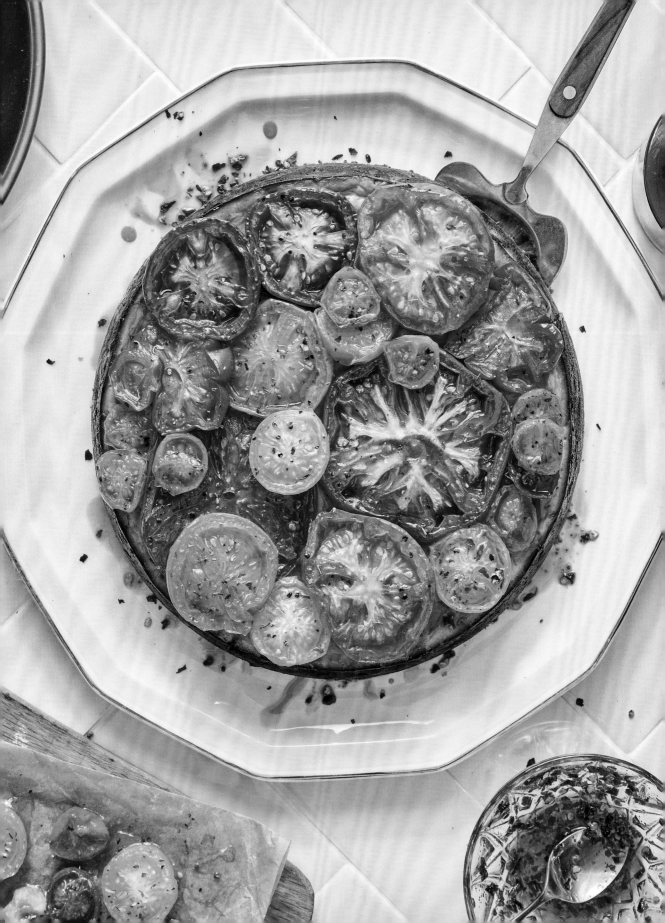

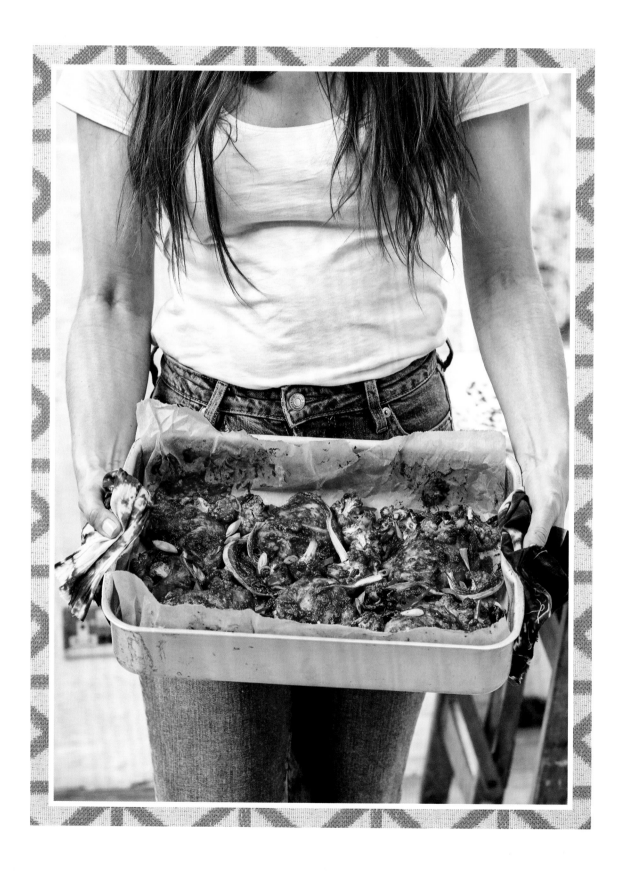

Chicken and cauliflower peanut sesame traybake Serves 2

Ingredients

4 organic bone-in chicken thighs

1 whole cauliflower (leaves and all), broken into bite-sized pieces

1 tablespoon sesame seeds (optional)

2 spring onions, sliced

1 red chilli, diced

salt and pepper

To serve

Serve with brown rice or quinoa

Marinade

3 tablespoons smooth peanut butter

1 tablespoon maple syrup or honey

4 tablespoons soy sauce or tamari

4 garlic cloves, crushed

thumb-sized piece of fresh ginger, skin on and grated

2 spring onions, finely chopped

1 red chilli, finely chopped

2 tablespoons extra virgin olive oil

Method

1. Preheat the oven to 180°C/160°C fan/350°F/ gas mark 4.

2. Make the marinade by mixing all the ingredients together in a bowl.

3. Score the chicken through the skin three times (this allows the marinade to seep in and speeds up cooking time).

4. Place the chicken and cauliflower on a lined baking tray and coat thoroughly with the marinade, using your hands if you need to, and (if you can) leave for 30 minutes. Sprinkle with sesame seeds, if using, season with pepper, then roast in the oven for 30–45 minutes.

5. Remove from the oven and scatter over the spring onions and chilli. Serve with brown rice or quinoa.

Cajun cod with black bean salsa Serves 2

Ingredients

2 teaspoons Cajun spice mix

juice of ½ lime

1 teaspoon honey

2 cod fillets (or any kind of white fish), skin off or on, whichever you prefer

salt and pepper

To serve

Serve with roasted sweet potato and steamed broccoli

Salsa

400g (14oz) can black beans, drained and rinsed

1 banana shallot, diced

6 cherry tomatoes, diced

2 teaspoons freshly chopped coriander

1 avocado, chopped

juice of 1 lime

1 tablespoon extra virgin olive oil

1 red chilli, finely chopped

Method

1. Preheat the oven to 200°C/180°C fan/400°F/ gas mark 6.

2. Mix the Cajun spice, lime juice and honey together in a bowl and then coat the cod fillets with this mixture. Season with salt and pepper and roast for 8–10 minutes.

3. Meanwhile, mix the salsa ingredients together and set aside.

4. Serve the Cajun cod and salsa with a roasted sweet potato and steamed broccoli.

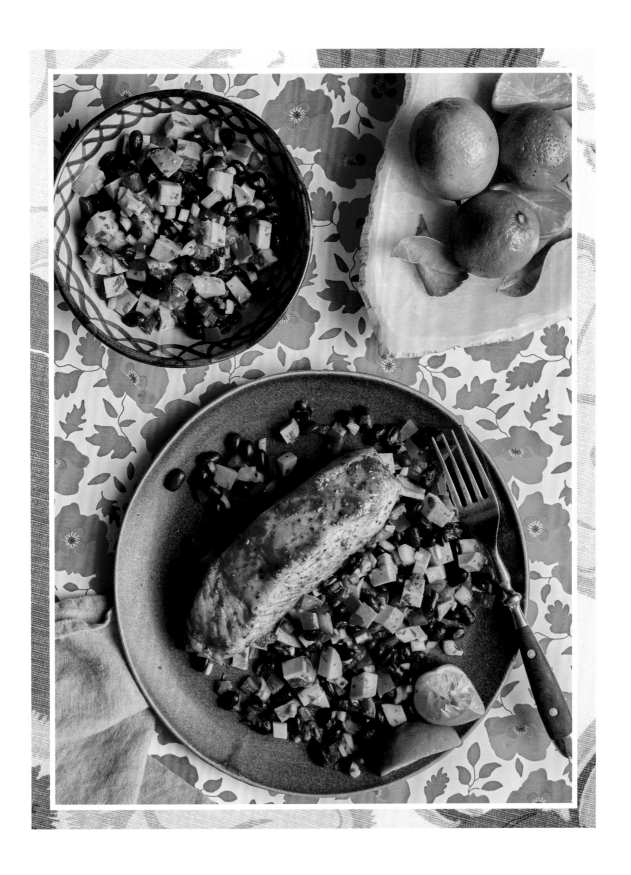

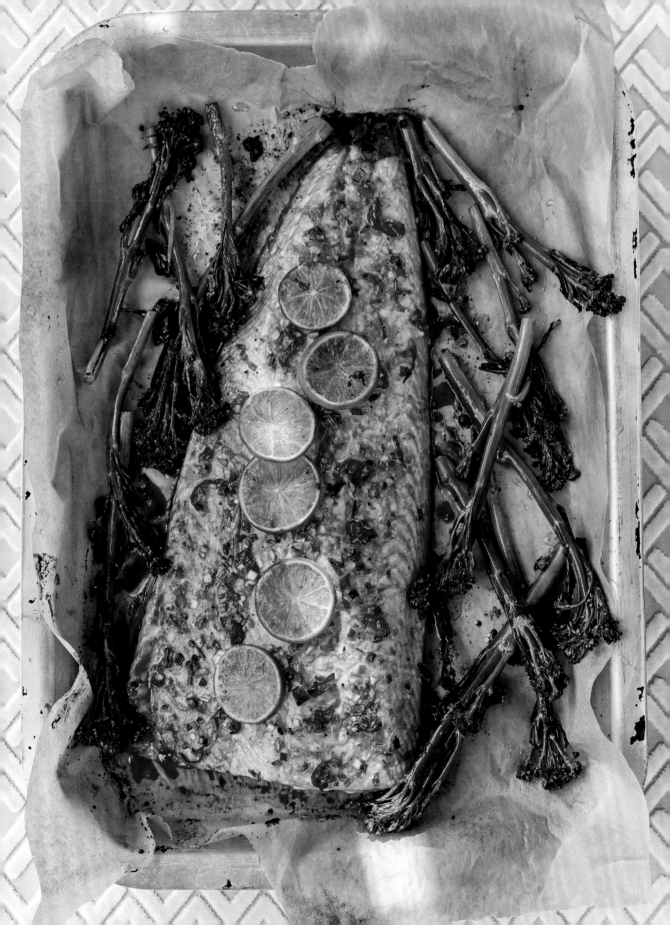

Soy and chilli salmon traybake Serves 4

Ingredients

4 salmon fillets, skin off or on, whichever you prefer

coriander, finely chopped

Marinade

2 garlic cloves, crushed

3 spring onions, finely chopped

1 tablespoon freshly grated ginger

1 red chilli, diced

2 tablespoons mirin

2 tablespoons Japanese rice wine vinegar

2 tablespoons light soy sauce or tamari

4 tablespoons extra virgin olive oil

salt and pepper

To serve

Serve with brown wholegrain rice or rice noodles and some steamed sugar snap peas or long-stem broccoli

Method

1. Preheat the oven to 200°C/180°C fan/400°F/gas mark 6.

2. Mix all the marinade ingredients together in a large bowl. Coat the salmon in the marinade and leave for 20 minutes.

3. Wrap the salmon and marinade in baking paper and fold closed so the salmon is covered, then cook in the oven for 10 minutes.

4. Serve with brown wholegrain rice or rice noodles and some steamed sugar snap peas or long-stem broccoli, and top with fresh coriander.

Fish pie with sweet potato mash Serves 2

Ingredients

400–450g (14oz–1lb) sweet potato, skin on and chopped into 2cm (¾in) pieces

extra virgin olive oil, for frying

2 leeks, thinly sliced with roots and ends removed

200ml (7fl oz) coconut milk

2 teaspoons cornflour

1 teaspoon smoked paprika

2 teaspoons wholegrain mustard

1 handful of fresh flat-leaf parsley, roughly chopped, plus extra to serve

½ teaspoon chilli flakes

300g (10½oz) fish pie selection (I like to use salmon and monkfish)

100g (3½oz) baby spinach

80g (2¾oz) green beans, trimmed

salt and pepper

To serve

Serve with steamed green beans

Method

1. Preheat the oven to 180°C/160°C fan/350°F/gas mark 4.

2. Place the sweet potato in a saucepan, cover with boiling water, bring to a simmer and cook for around 5 minutes until soft. Drain and set aside.

3. Place another pan over a medium heat and add some extra virgin olive oil. Add the leeks and cook for 5 minutes.

4. Pour 1 tablespoon of coconut milk into a bowl and mix with the cornflour to form a smooth paste. Add the remaining coconut milk to the leeks along with the cornflour paste, smoked paprika, mustard, parsley and chilli flakes and season with salt and pepper. Simmer gently for 5 minutes until the sauce thickens.

5. Place the leek mixture into a baking dish, then stir through the fish mix. Stir in the spinach.

6. Mash the sweet potato with some extra virgin olive oil and salt and pepper.

7. Spoon the mash over the fish and place in the fridge until ready to cook, or bake in the oven for 15–20 minutes.

8. Serve the fish pie with steamed green beans and top with the remaining parsley. Then enjoy!

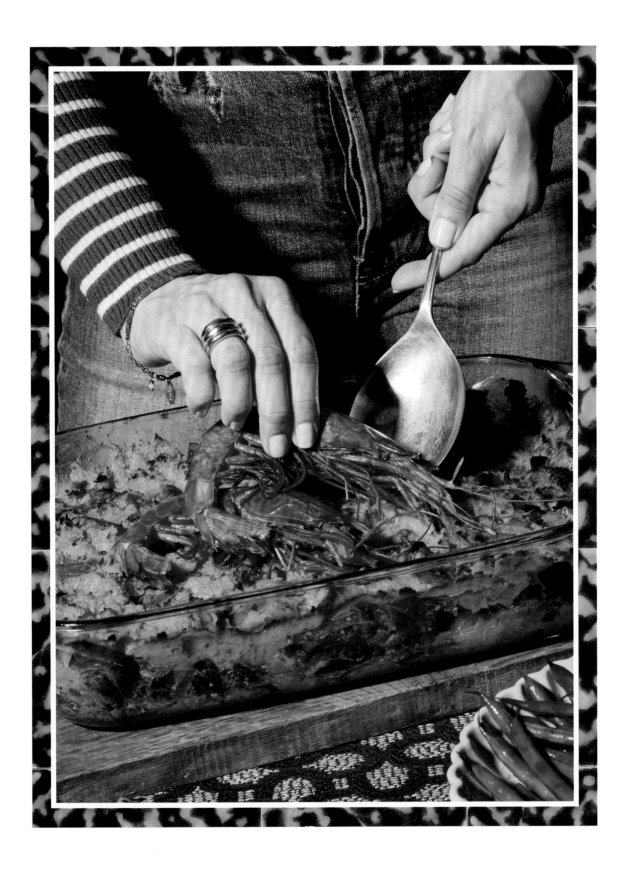

Desserts & sweet things

Brown rice pudding Serves 2

Ingredients

200g (1 cup) brown rice

400ml (14fl oz) coconut milk

1 teaspoon maple syrup
(depending on how sweet you
like things)

1 teaspoon ground cinnamon

4 tablespoons raisins

½ vanilla pod, scraped,
or ½ teaspoon vanilla
essence (optional)

To serve

Serve with ice cream or
natural yogurt and freshly
grated nutmeg

Method

1. Rinse the brown rice under cold water for about
   10 seconds then place in a pan and cover with
   cold water so there is about 2.5cm (1in) of water
   above the rice. Place over a medium heat, bring
   to the boil and simmer until the rice is cooked
   (about 35 minutes).

2. Remove from the heat, cover and set aside for
   10 minutes, then stir.

3. Pour in the coconut milk and add the maple
   syrup, cinnamon and raisins. Simmer, uncovered,
   stirring frequently, for 20 minutes or until your
   desired consistency is reached.

4. Remove from the heat and stir in the vanilla.

5. Top with ice cream or yogurt and nutmeg to serve.

Easy apple pie Serves 1

Ingredients

1 tablespoon coconut oil

2 apples, cored and chopped
into 2cm (¾in) cubes

½ teaspoon nutmeg

½ teaspoon ground cinnamon

1 tablespoon maple syrup

45g (½ cup) 100 per cent
rolled oats

juice of ½ lemon

To serve

Serve with natural yogurt
and basil or Greek basil

Method

1. Melt the coconut oil in a pan. Add the apples,
   nutmeg, cinnamon, maple syrup, oats and
   lemon juice, then cook, stirring regularly, for
   about 5 minutes.

2. Place in a bowl and top with yogurt and basil
   or Greek basil if you fancy. Enjoy!

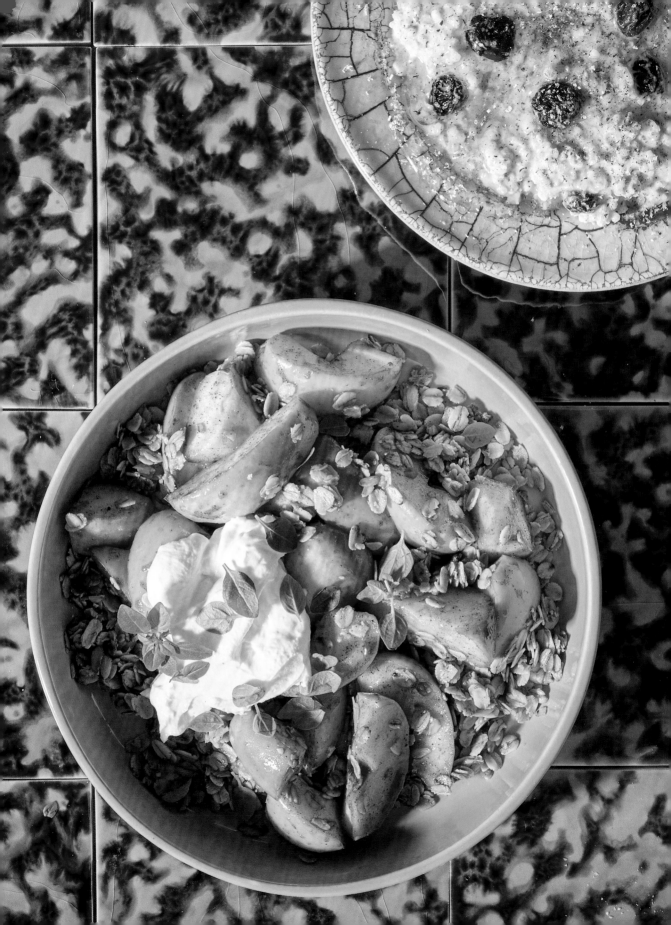

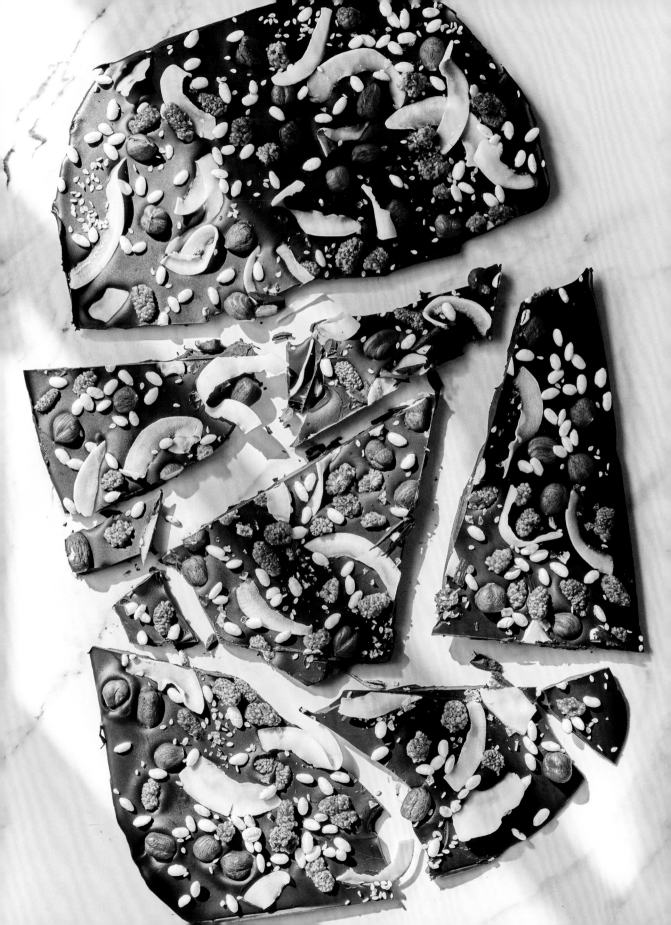

Dark chocolate bark Serves 4–5

Ingredients

2 x 100g (3½oz) bars of dark chocolate (I use the brand Lindt 70 per cent)

1 tsp extra virgin olive oil

Toppings

seeds, such as flaxseeds, chia seeds, hemp seeds or sunflower seeds

mixed nuts

dried mulberries

puffed rice

dried coconut flakes

Method

1. Melt the dark chocolate in the microwave in 30-second bursts, stirring after each one. The chocolate is done when it's about 90 per cent melted, keep stirring and the residual heat should melt the remaining pieces.

2. Stir in the extra virgin olive oil.

3. Pour the mixture onto a lined baking tray. Using a silicone or rubber spatula, spread the chocolate evenly over the centre area of the baking tray – aim for a thickness of about 5mm (¼in) – it won't reach the edges.

4. Sprinkle the seeds, mixed nuts, dried mulberries, puffed rice and coconut flakes evenly over the chocolate.

5. Place the tray on a flat surface in the fridge to harden for about 30 minutes (until firmly set), then remove and break into pieces. Enjoy! Store in an airtight container in the fridge for up to 2 months.

Fudgy tahini brownies Makes 9

Ingredients

4 tablespoons ground flaxseeds mixed with 10 tablespoons warm water (or 2 free-range organic eggs)

about 2 big bananas, mashed

120g (1/2 cup) smooth tahini

180g (3/4 cup) maple syrup

40g (1/2 cup) oat flour

50g (1 cup) cacao powder

¼ teaspoon salt

chocolate chips of your choice

Method

1. First make the flax eggs in a small bowl by combining the ground flaxseeds with the water, then set aside.

2. Preheat the oven to 180°C/160°C fan/350°F/gas mark 4 and line a 20cm (8in) square baking tin with baking parchment.

3. Add the mashed bananas to a bowl together with the tahini, maple syrup and flax eggs. Whisk until fully combined and smooth.

4. Fold in the oat flour, cacao powder and salt. Pour the batter into the prepared tin and bake for 35 minutes.

5. When the brownies are done, add the chocolate chips on top, let them melt and then spread evenly on top.

6. Leave the brownies to cool in the tin for about 15 minutes before serving. Store in an airtight container in the fridge for up to 1 week.

Tip: Serve the brownies warm with vanilla banana nice cream (blended frozen banana) on top.

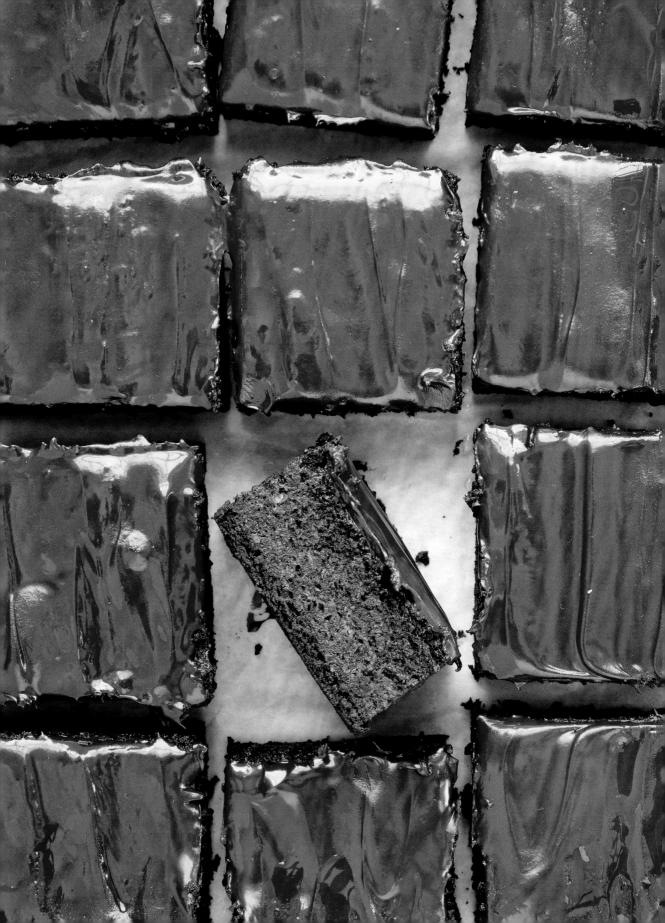

Fudgy flourless mug cake Makes 1 mug cake

Ingredients

1 banana, mashed

2 tablespoons cacao powder

2 tablespoons smooth
peanut butter

2 tablespoons dairy-free
choc chips

Method

1. Mix all the ingredients together in a mug and place in the microwave on full power for 2 minutes.

The best blondies
(gluten- and dairy-free) Makes about 9 blondies

Ingredients

180g (1½ cups) almond flour

¼ teaspoon bicarbonate
of soda

60g (⅓ cup) coconut sugar
(or any kind of sugar you like)

pinch of salt

25g (¼ cup) coconut oil, melted

2 tablespoons almond milk

2 eggs

1 teaspoon pure vanilla extract

dairy-free mini chocolate chips

Method

1. Preheat the oven to 180°C/160°C/350°F/gas mark 4.

2. Grab your food processer and pop in the almond flour, bicarbonate of soda, coconut sugar and salt.

3. In a separate bowl, add the melted coconut oil, almond milk, eggs and vanilla extract, then whisk together.

4. Mix the dry ingredients together first, then add the wet ingredients to the food processor and mix it all together.

5. Next, stir in the chocolate chips, reserving a few for topping.

6. Line a baking tin with baking parchment, then pour in the blondie mixture, top with the reserved chocolate chips and bake for 25–30 minutes. When a knife inserted into the centre comes out clean, you're good to go. Don't forget to let them cool before you tuck in. Store in an airtight container in the fridge for up to 1 week.

Tip: If you would like it vegan, you can use flax eggs. Mix 2 tablespoons of ground flaxseeds with 6 tablespoons of warm water, stir and refrigerate until it sticks together. Follow the method as above but cook for 32 minutes.

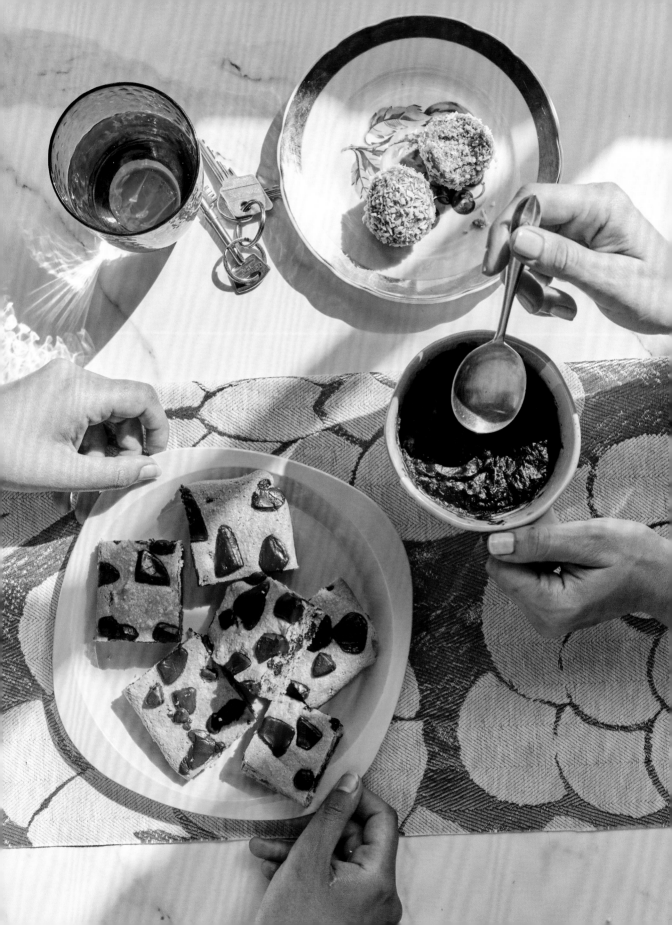

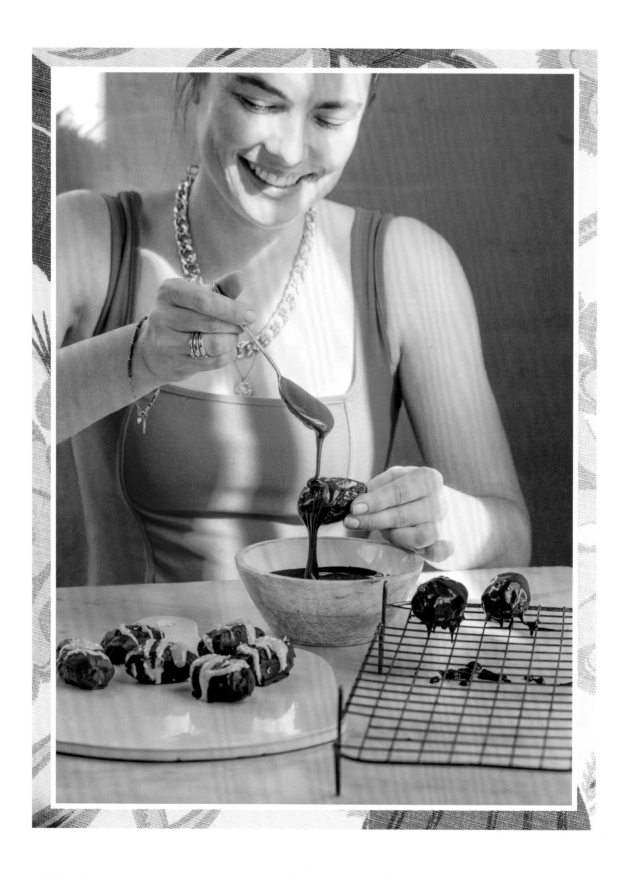

Chocolate and peanut date bites Makes 9

Ingredients

9 Medjool dates

280g (10oz) jar of peanut butter

about a palm-sized serving
of nuts of your choice
(I used hazelnuts)

200g (7oz) dark chocolate (at
least 70 per cent cocoa solids)

sea salt

Method

1. Place the dates on a chopping board and slice vertically, removing the stones as you go.

2. Spoon some of the peanut butter into the openings of each date.

3. Chop the nuts and then sprinkle them into the dates on top of the peanut butter.

4. Melt the chocolate and then dip each date into it. Make sure the dates are entirely covered, then transfer immediately to a cooling rack.

5. When all the dates are covered in chocolate, pop them in the fridge on the rack, with a plate underneath, for around 30 minutes.

6. Once the chocolate has cooled, remove the dates from the fridge, drizzle with the remaining peanut butter and sprinkle with sea salt. Enjoy!

Tiny chocolate tahini cookies Makes 24

Ingredients

1 tablespoon ground flaxseed mixed with 3 tablespoons warm water (or 1 free-range organic egg)

120g (½ cup) tahini

110g (½ cup) maple syrup

75g (¾ cup) almond flour

50g (½ cup) unsweetened cocoa powder

45g (¼ cup) coconut sugar or any kind of sugar

½ teaspoon baking powder

½ teaspoon bicarbonate of soda

½ teaspoon salt

1 teaspoon vanilla extract

85g (½ cup) dairy-free chocolate chips

35–70g (¼–½ cup) sesame seeds

1 teaspoon sea salt

olive oil, for greasing

Method

1. Combine the flaxseed and warm water to make the flax egg and set aside for 2 minutes. Line a baking sheet with baking parchment.

2. In a large bowl, whisk together the tahini, maple syrup and flax egg (or egg, if using). Add the almond flour, cocoa powder, sugar, baking powder, bicarbonate of soda, salt and vanilla extract and stir until fully combined. Fold in the chocolate chips. Cover the bowl with clingfilm (or similar) and chill in the fridge for at least 1 hour.

3. Preheat the oven to 180°C/160°C fan/350°F/gas mark 4. Place the sesame seeds and sea salt in a small bowl and stir to combine. Fill another small bowl with water. The cookie dough will be sticky, so rub your hands with some olive oil, then, using a small spoon, scoop a spoonful of cookie dough and gently roll it into a loose ball with your hands. Repeat with the remaining dough.

4. Dip or roll each cookie in the sesame salt and place on the prepared baking sheet. Dip a fork into the water and press down slightly vertically and then horizontally on top of each cookie. Dip the fork in the water every time. This is to make sure the cookies spread out into even circles during baking.

5. Bake for 10–12 minutes. Remove from the oven and wait a minute or two before transferring to a wire rack to cool. Store in an airtight container for up to 2 weeks.

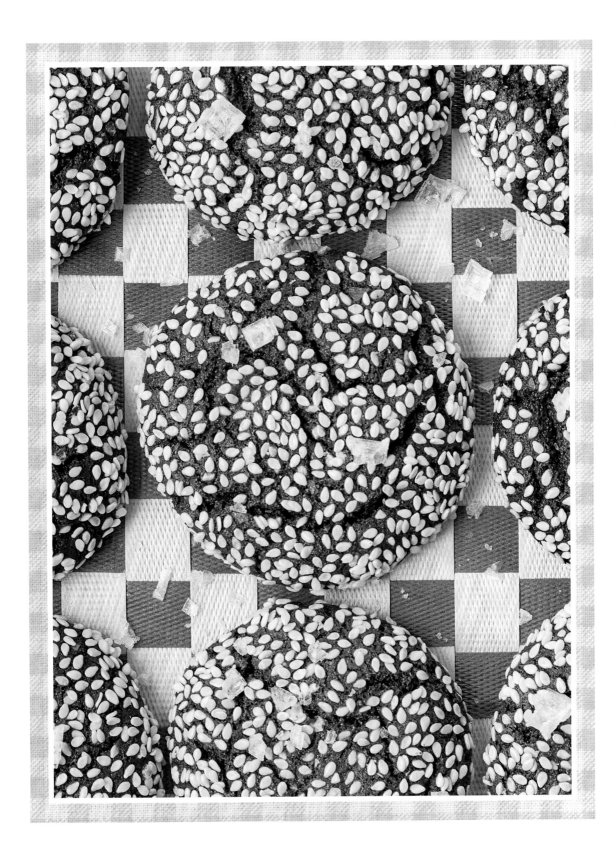

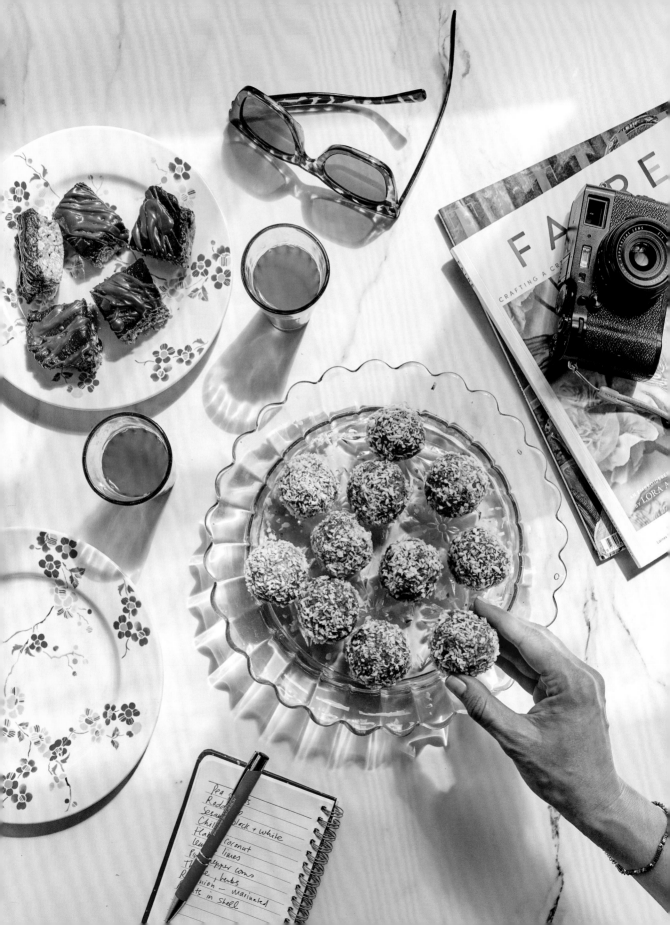

Chocolate flapjack bites Makes 9 bites

Ingredients

180g (6oz) 100 per cent rolled oats

5 tablespoons desiccated coconut

250g (9oz) smooth peanut butter

230g (8oz) honey or maple syrup

Topping

12 Medjool dates, pitted

60g (2¼oz) cacao powder

7 tablespoons coconut oil, melted

2 tablespoons coconut milk

1 teaspoon maple syrup

Method

1. Start by making the base. Mix the oats, coconut, peanut butter and honey or maple syrup together in a large mixing bowl. (You may need to heat the honey slightly if it is not very runny.)

2. Line a 20cm (8in) square baking tin with baking parchment and push the mixture evenly down into it. Set aside in the fridge.

3. Next, make the topping by placing all the ingredients in a food processor and blending until smooth.

4. Spoon the topping evenly over the base. You may also like to melt some dark chocolate and drizzle it over the top. Then pop this all back in the fridge for at least 1 hour.

5. Store in an airtight container in the fridge for up to 2 weeks.

The best energy balls Makes 12

Ingredients

12 Medjool dates, pitted

4 tablespoons smooth nut butter of your choice (I used peanut butter)

100g (1 cup) ground almonds

95g (1 cup) desiccated coconut, plus extra for rolling

2 tablespoons maca powder

pinch of salt

honey, for rolling

Method

1. Pop the dates and nut butter into a food processor and blend to a paste.

2. Add in the remaining ingredients and blend until combined.

3. Shape into 3cm (1¼in) balls, then roll in honey, followed by desiccated coconut. Store in the fridge in an airtight container for up to 2 weeks.

Matcha cheesecake

Makes about 6–8 slices

Ingredients

120g (1½ cups) 100 per cent
rolled oats

225g (1½ cups) whole almonds

¼ teaspoon sea salt

4 tablespoons coconut sugar

4–6 tablespoons coconut oil,
melted, plus extra for greasing

Filling

about 300g (10½oz) silken tofu

165g (⅔ cup) full-fat
coconut milk

zest and juice of 2 lemons

4 tablespoons coconut sugar

2 tablespoons arrowroot

4 teaspoons pure
vanilla extract

2 tablespoons matcha green
tea powder, plus extra to serve

To serve

Raspberries and coconut
flakes, to garnish (optional)

Method

1. Preheat the oven to 180°C/160°C fan/350°F/gas mark 4.

2. Start by making the base. Grab your food processor and add the oats, almonds, salt, coconut sugar and melted coconut oil. Blend until you have a soft, sticky dough – you may need to add 1–2 tablespoons more melted coconut oil.

3. Grease a 23cm (9in) springform cake tin with coconut oil.

4. Press the dough into the tin, extending it about 2.5cm (1in) up the sides. Poke the base with a fork a few times and bake for 25 minutes until brown and crispy.

5. To make the filling, place the silken tofu, coconut milk, lemon zest and juice, coconut sugar, arrowroot and vanilla extract in a food processor and blend. Next, sift the matcha into the silken tofu mixture, and blend again.

6. Pour the mixture into the cooked crust, then tap on the work surface 3–4 times to remove any air bubbles. Bake for a further 25–30 minutes until the top is golden brown.

7. Let the cheesecake cool at room temperature for 30 minutes, then pop in the fridge for 2–3 hours.

8. Sift over some extra matcha powder to serve. Dress with sliced lemons, raspberries and coconut flakes, if you like.

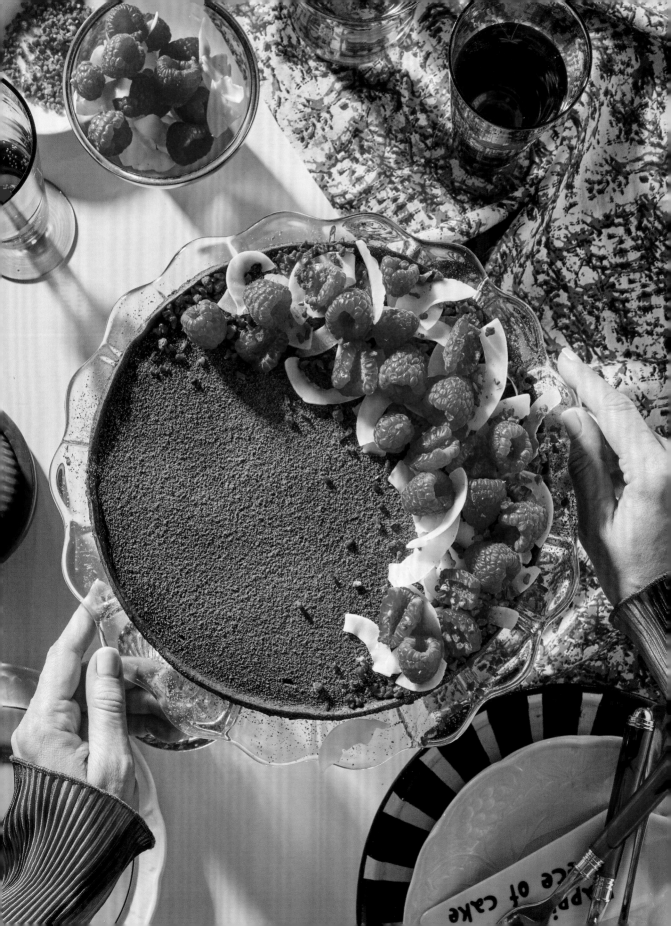

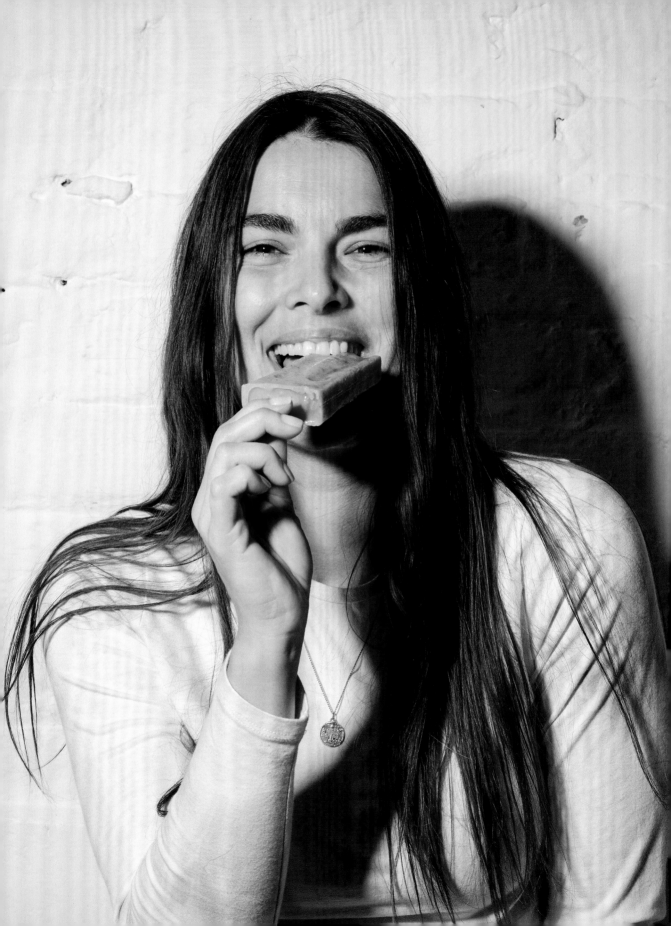

Synbiotic strawberry lollies

Makes 5 lollies, depending on the size of your mould

Ingredients

200g (7oz) strawberries, hulled

1 ripe banana

2 Medjool dates, chopped
and mixed with 1 tablespoon
boiling water

100g (3½oz) live full-fat yogurt
(dairy or coconut)

Method

1. Place all the ingredients in a blender and roughly blend, then transfer one-third of the mixture to a bowl.

2. Blend the remaining mixture until smooth, then add to the mixture in the bowl and stir to combine.

3. Spoon into ice-lolly moulds and place in the freezer for at least 4 hours or until solid.

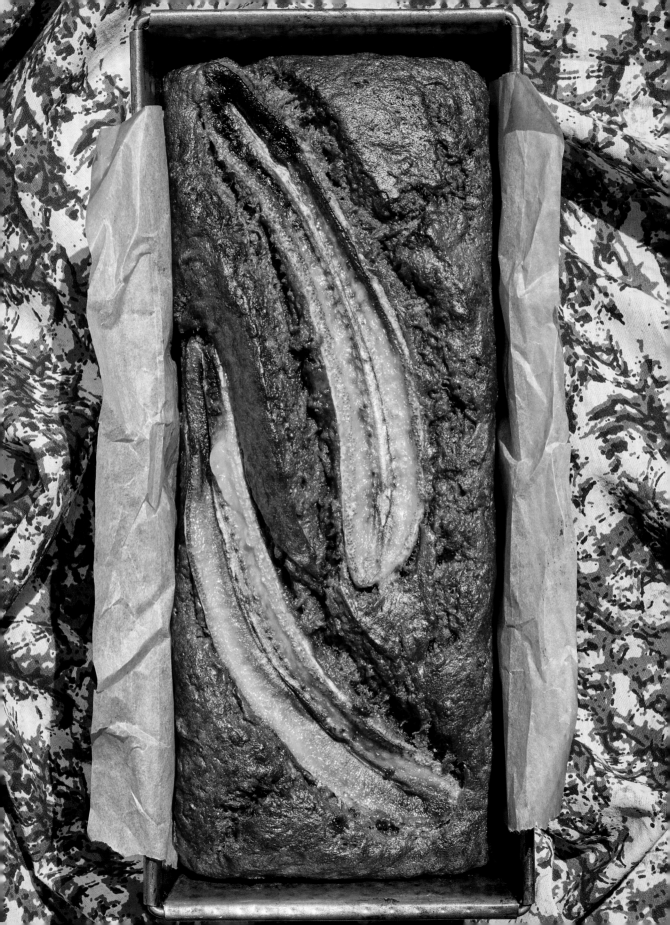

Cocoa banana bread Serves 8–12

Ingredients

225g (8oz) plain flour

1 tablespoon unsweetened cocoa powder

1 teaspoon bicarbonate of soda

1 teaspoon salt

90g (3¼oz) coconut oil, melted, plus extra for greasing

175g (6oz) light brown sugar, plus extra for sprinkling

1 teaspoon natural vanilla extract

1 large organic, free-range egg

5 extremely ripe bananas, 4 roughly mashed and 1 cut lengthwise

125g (4½oz) full-fat yogurt

Method

1. Preheat your oven to 180°C/160°C fan/350°F/gas mark 4. Grab a 23 x 10cm (9 x 4in) loaf tin and grease with some coconut oil.

2. In a bowl, whisk together the flour, cocoa powder, bicarbonate of soda and salt.

3. In a separate bowl, add the coconut oil, sugar and vanilla and beat for 3–5 minutes with (ideally) an electric whisk until the mixture is light and fluffy. Scrape down the sides of the bowl and add the egg. Beat for about 2 minutes until well combined and the mixture is light and fluffy.

4. Slowly add the dry ingredients to the wet and mix to combine.

5. Using a spatula or wooden spoon, fold in the mashed banana, followed by the yogurt and mix together.

6. Pour the batter into the prepared loaf tin, smoothing the top. Place the banana halves, cut-side up, on top of the batter and sprinkle the entire top with some extra sugar.

7. Bake for 1½ hours–1 hour 40 minutes until the sides have started to come away from the tin and the centre is cooked.

8. Leave to cool, then enjoy. Keep stored in an airtight container at room temperature for 3–4 days or in the fridge for up to a week.

Raspberry mousse Serves 4

Ingredients

450g (1lb) raspberries

1 avocado

1 vanilla pod, scraped out

1 tablespoon honey
or maple syrup

3 tablespoons almond butter

100g (3½oz) coconut cream

Method

1. Pop all the ingredients in a blender, reserving some of the raspberries for topping, and blend until smooth.

2. Decant into 4 glasses, top with the reserved rapsberries and place in the fridge for at least 1 hour. Then you're ready to serve.

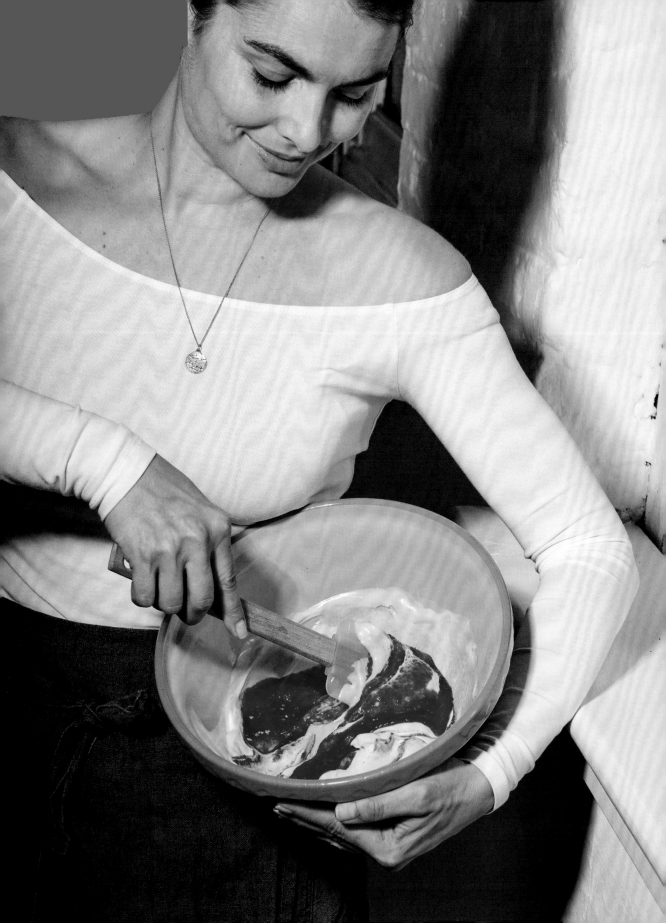

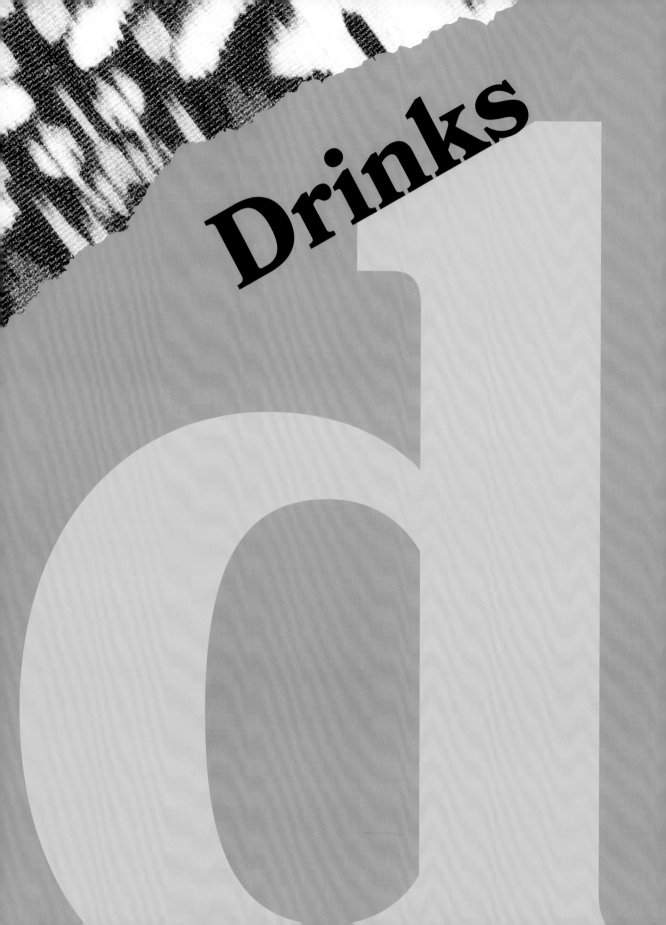

Drinks

d1

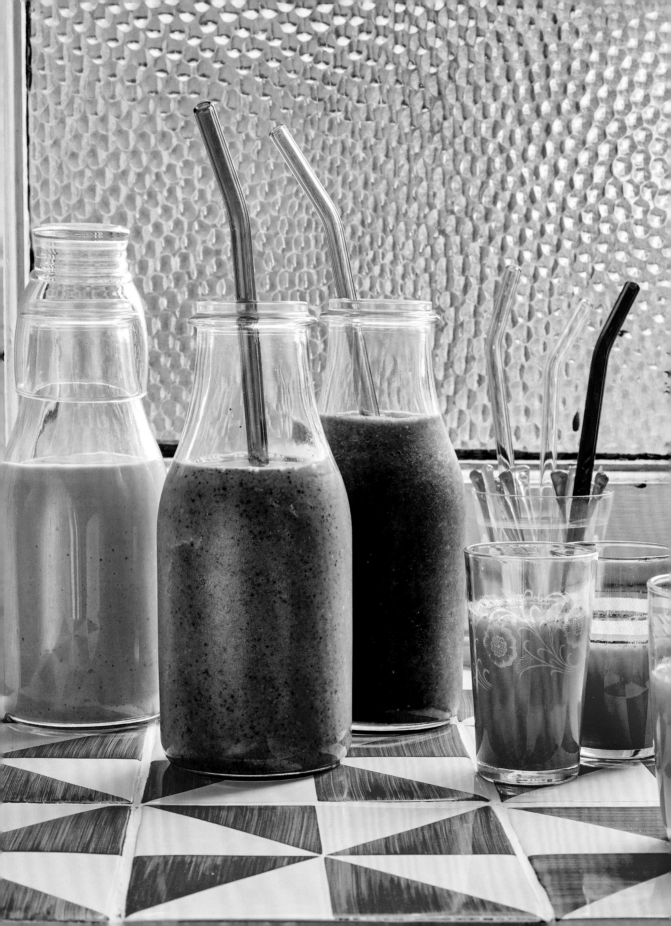

Smoothies and hot shot

Breakfast smoothie Serves 2

200ml (7fl oz) milk of your choice

50ml (about 3–4 tablespoons) kefir or yogurt

1 tablespoon nut butter of your choice

1 small avocado

1 small handful of raspberries or blueberries

½ tablespoon 100 per cent cacao powder

¼ teaspoon ground cinnamon

½ teaspoon ground turmeric (optional)

Place all the ingredients in a blender and blend until smooth. Divide between two glasses and enjoy!

Blueberry boost smoothie Serves 1

150g (5½oz) blueberries (fresh or frozen)

½ avocado

2 handfuls of leafy greens, such as spinach or kale (fresh or frozen)

1 handful of walnuts

150ml (5fl oz) milk of your choice

Place all the ingredients in a blender and blend until smooth.

My favourite green smoothie Serves 2

300ml (10fl oz) milk of your choice

1 banana, frozen

½ cucumber (can be frozen)

1 kiwi, skin on or off, whichever you prefer

1 large handful (100g) of dark leafy greens, such as spinach, kale, Swiss chard

1 teaspoon hemp or chia seeds

1 tablespoon nut butter of your choice

1 tablespoon protein powder (optional)

Place all the ingredients in a blender and blend until smooth. Divide between two glasses and enjoy!

Hot turmeric shot Makes 4–6 shots

thumb-sized piece of fresh ginger, sliced

juice of 1 lemon

½ teaspoon ground turmeric

½ garlic clove

grind of pepper

1 teaspoon honey

235ml (1 cup) boiling water

Place all the ingredients in a blender cup and blend until smooth. Watch for spitting when you open the cup after blending. Then pour into shot glasses or small glasses and enjoy!

Pomegranate, ginger and mint cooler Makes about 4 glasses

Ingredients

½ pomegranate

2cm (¾in) piece of fresh ginger, peeled

1 handful of fresh mint leaves

Method

1. Hold the pomegranate cut-side down in your fingers and bash the back of it with a spoon so the seeds tumble into a jug.

2. Finely grate in some ginger, then add the mint.

3. Add loads of ice, then top up with water and leave to infuse for at least 1 hour. Pour into glasses, then enjoy.

Rooibos and thyme iced tea Serves 4

Ingredients

85g (1/4 cup) honey

6 slices of fresh ginger, peeled (each 1/4in thick), plus extra to serve

1 bunch of fresh thyme

3 limes: juice of 2, 1 quartered, plus slices to serve

700ml (1¼ pints) rooibos tea, chilled (or you can use black tea if you can't find rooibos)

Method

1. Combine the honey, ginger, eight thyme sprigs and quartered lime in a cocktail shaker. Shake until the lime quarters release their juices and the ginger and thyme begin to break down.

2. Add the lime juice, stirring until the honey has completely dissolved. Strain the mixture into a pitcher partially filled with ice or divide evenly between four ice-filled glasses.

3. Top with the tea, stirring to evenly combine. Garnish with thyme sprigs, ginger slices and lime slices, then enjoy!

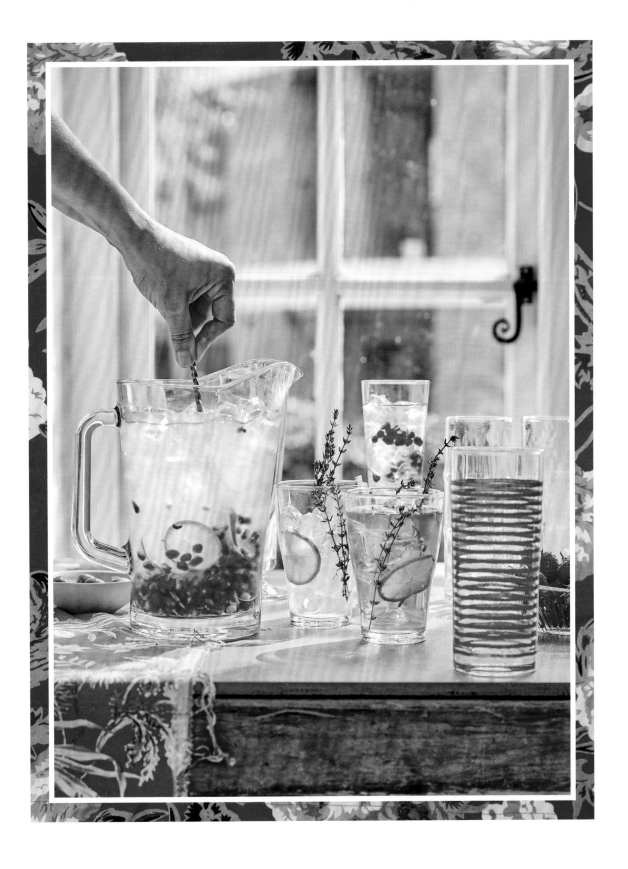

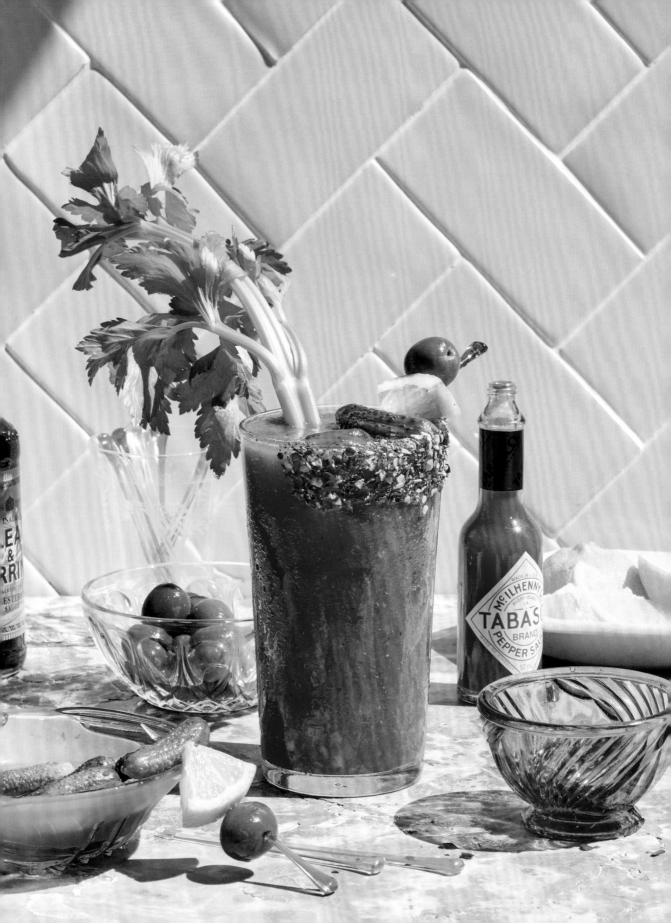

Ultimate Virgin Mary Makes about 4–6 glasses

Ingredients

1 litre (1¾ pints) tomato juice

1 medium–large cucumber, peeled and seeded

juice of 3 lemons, plus lemon slices to serve

1 teaspoon celery seed (not celery salt)

1 teaspoon Worcestershire sauce

½ teaspoon hot sauce (I use Tabasco), plus extra to taste

1 teaspoon (about 50 twists) freshly ground black pepper

2 medium garlic cloves, crushed

¼ teaspoon celery salt (optional)

lots of ice, to serve

Garnishes
(choose any)

celery stalks, cucumber sticks, dill pickle spears, and/or green olives

Method

1. In a blender, combine the tomato juice, cucumber, lemon juice, celery seed, Worcestershire sauce and hot sauce. Securely fasten the lid and blend on high speed until completely smooth.

2. Taste, and add more hot sauce for more heat. If you like, then add the black pepper and garlic. Securely fasten the lid and blend for just a few seconds. Add celery salt to taste.

3. Fill your glasses with ice and pour the Virgin Mary mix over the top. Stir with a spoon, garnish with a slice of lemon and then serve immediately.

Chocolate and
hazelnut milkshake Serves 1

Ingredients

1–2 frozen bananas

1 tablespoon smooth
peanut butter

200ml (7fl oz) nut milk

1–2 teaspoons melted chocolate

1 palm-sized serving of
hazlenuts, chopped/crushed

pinch of cacao nibs

Method

1. Blend the bananas, peanut butter, milk and melted chocolate, reserving
    a small amount of the latter.

2. Drizzle the reserved chocolate around the inside of the cup and fill with
    your blended mixture.

3. Top with crushed hazelnuts and cacao nibs. Enjoy!

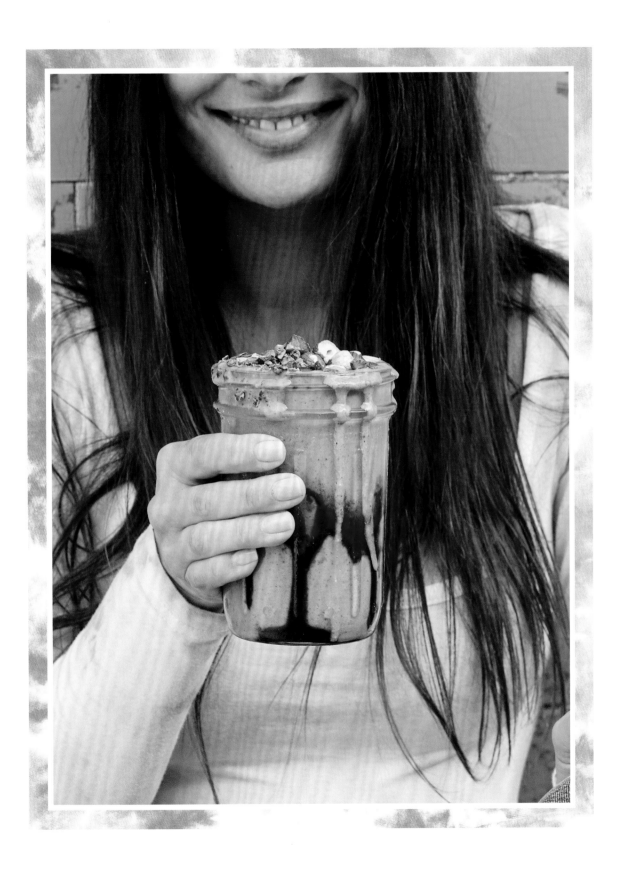

Rosemary grapefruit fizz Makes 6–8 glasses

Ingredients

500ml (18fl oz) grapefruit juice

4 tablespoons rosemary
sugar syrup (see below)

1 litre sparkling water

sliced grapefruit

ice cubes

Rosemary sugar syrup

250ml (9fl oz) water

200g (7oz) sugar
(I used white table sugar)

6 sprigs of rosemary fresh,
plus extra to serve

Method

1. If you don't have store-bought grapefruit juice, start with juicing them. You'll need about six grapefruits.

2. To make the rosemary sugar syrup, place the filtered water in a pan and bring to the boil, then add the sugar and stir to dissolve. Add the rosemary and let the infusion boil for 1 minute. Remove the pan from the heat and let it seep for 30 minutes–1 hour, depending on how strong you would like it. Pour the cooled syrup through a mesh strainer into an airtight container, preferably glass. This can be stored in the fridge for up to 2 weeks.

3. To make the drink, grab a jug and add the grapefruit juice and rosemary syrup. Stir, then top with sparkling water to your desired strength, and stir again. Enjoy immediately or keep in the fridge.

4. When you're ready to serve, place rosemary sprigs, slices of grapefruit, and ice cubes into a glass then pour over your grapefruit fizz.

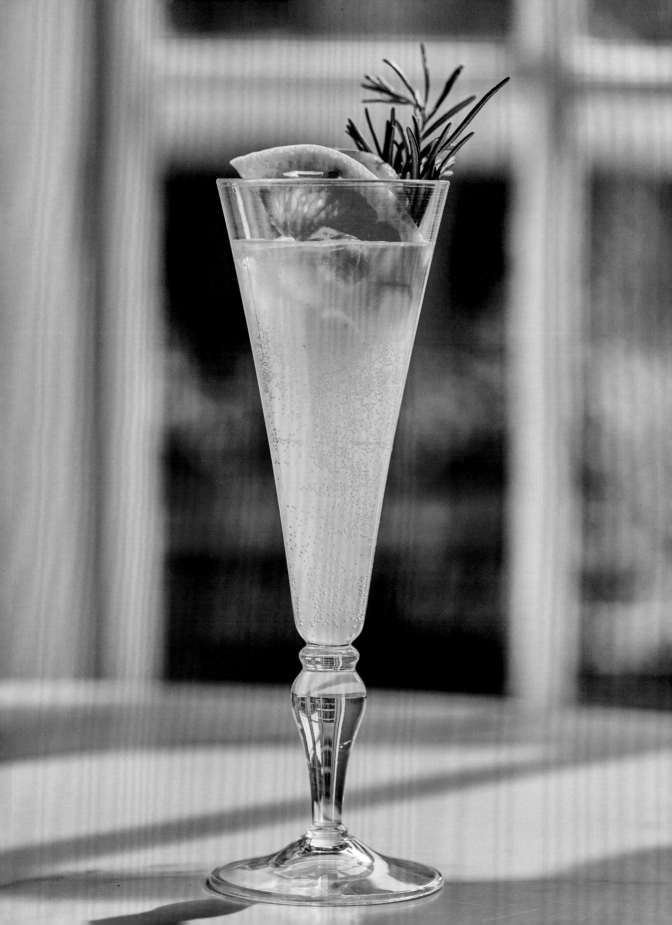

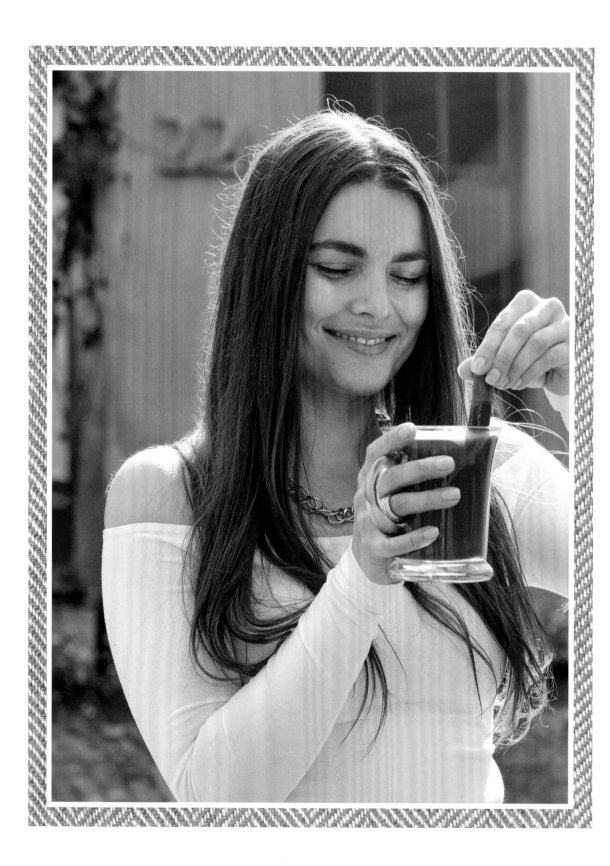

Snuggle-down spiced hot chocolate Serves 2

Ingredients

400ml (14fl oz) milk of your choice

3 tablespoons cacao powder

1½ tablespoons maple syrup or honey

1 teaspoon ground cinnamon

pinch of cayenne pepper (optional)

Method

1. Whisk all the ingredients together and warm gently in a saucepan before pouring into mugs. Enjoy!

Cardamom and ginger chai spice tea Serves 2

Ingredients

500ml (2 cups) filtered water

thumb-sized piece of ginger, sliced lengthwise

4 cardamom pods and seeds, crushed

1 teaspoon Darjeeling or Assam tea leaves, to taste

2 tablespoons honey

250ml (1 cup) milk of your choice (I use almond milk)

Method

1. Place a small milk pan over a medium heat. Add the filtered water, ginger and crushed cardamom to the water and bring to the boil, then reduce to a simmer.

2. Simmer for 5–7 minutes until the colour of the water changes to a mild yellowish colour.

3. Add the tea leaves and simmer for about 3 minutes.

4. Next, add the honey and simmer for 2–3 minutes until the water turns a deep red and the sugar has dissolved. Simmering makes the tea stronger. If you prefer a light version, reduce the simmering time, and check the colour.

5. Finally, add the milk and simmer for a further 1–2 minutes.

6. Remove from the heat and strain the tea through a metal sieve, then pour into a cup and enjoy.

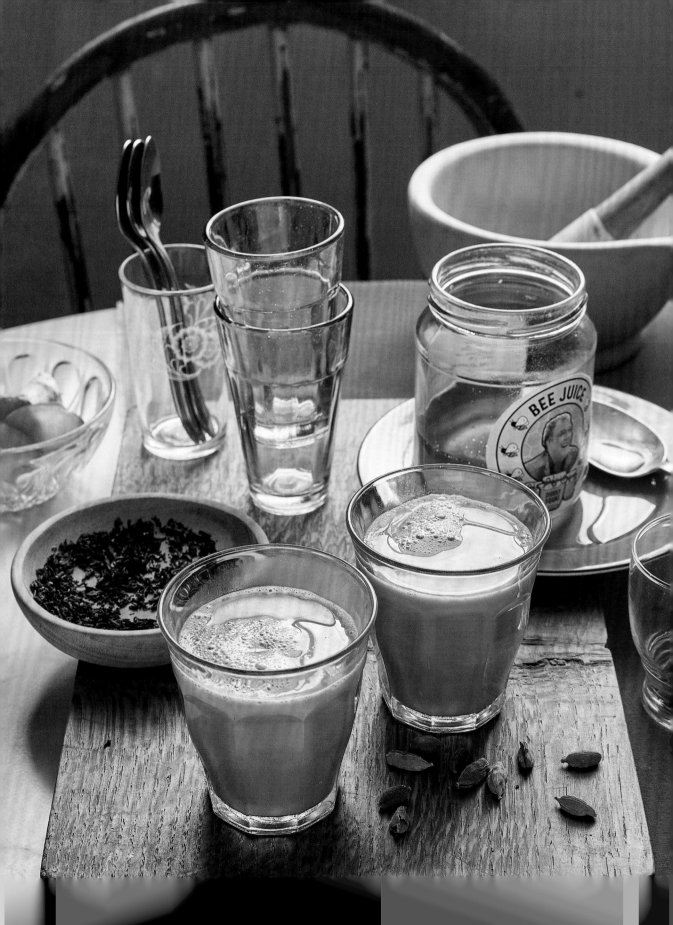

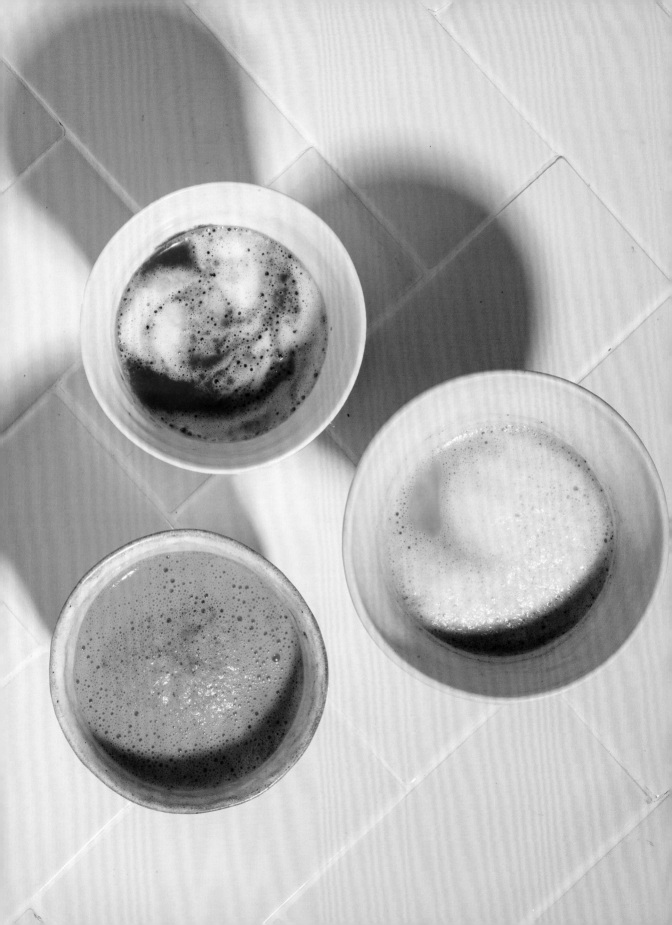

Lattes

Beetroot latte Serves 1

1 teaspoon beetroot powder

1 teaspoon maple syrup

250ml (1 cup) milk of
your choice

pinch of ground
ginger (optional)

1. Place all the ingredients in a pan over a medium heat and simmer
for 8–10 minutes.

2. Whisk for about 1 minute until some froth forms or use a milk frother
if you have one. Pour into a mug and enjoy.

Matcha green tea latte Serves 1

1 teaspoon matcha green
tea powder, plus extra to
serve (optional)

2 teaspoons honey
or maple syrup

3 tablespoons warm water

250–300ml (1–1¼ cups)
milk of your choice

1. Spoon the matcha green tea powder and honey or maple syrup into a mug or cup.

2. Add the warm water and mix with a spoon or with a whisk until it is a smooth,
dark green paste with no lumps.

3. If enjoying hot, warm 300ml (1¼ cups) milk in a small saucepan and pour
into the mug until nearly full. Use 250ml (1 cup) cold milk for an iced latte.

4. Use a whisk to mix the paste and milk together until smooth and light
green in colour.

5. If serving hot, you might like to add a few sprinkles of matcha green tea powder on
top for decoration. If serving cold, pour over ice cubes for an extra-cold iced latte.

Turmeric latte Serves 1

½–1 teaspoon ground turmeric

½ teaspoon ground ginger

½ teaspoon ground cinnamon

½ teaspoon maple syrup

200ml (scant 1 cup) milk of
your choice

grind of pepper

1. Place all the ingredients in a pan over a medium heat, then simmer for
8–10 minutes, whisking constantly, or use a milk frother if you have one.

2. Once hot, pour into a mug and enjoy!

Acknowledgements

To my parents who have sacrificed so much for me and without whom I wouldn't be where I am today. I will forever be grateful for everything you have done for me and I love you both very much.

To my agent Adrian who believed in me from the first moment we met. I am enormously thankful for your cheerleading, straight-talking guidance and general handholding.

To Judith for believing in this project and trusting my vision, and to the rest of the Kyle team. Especially the brilliant Emma for her enthusiasm and patience. Joanna, Victoria and Charlotte, thank you for your overwhelming support and for sharing my passion.

To Lucy and Ellen at Imagist for your insanely hard work, long hours, wonderfully upbeat attitudes and incredible talent. Thank you for understanding what I wanted to create even when the only place it existed at the time was in my head.

To Nick and Vanessa, two of the kindest and most creative people I know. Nick, thank you for your willingness and enthusiasm taking on this project, and injecting your talent and magic into it. And to Vanessa for bringing my vision to life; I couldn't have done it without you, and your positive creative influence helped me to go further then I knew I could. To Kristine, thank you for your immense hard work and unbelievable cooking. And to Lucy and Holly, thank you for your cheerful attitudes and for all your help along the way.

For the gorgeous backgrounds that were lent especially my super talented friend Octavia Dickinson and Balineum tiles.

To Tallulah for starting me on the journey.

To Amy for so generously giving up her time and wisdom over the years, as well as sparking my passion for photography.

To Tom for your unbelievable kindness, thoughtfulness and support, even when you didn't have to.

To Drew for inspiring and guiding me. Thank you for explaining the world of video making to me and igniting my love of videography.

To Carrie for hanging and crouching in almost every position imaginable to help me to get my lifestyle shots. Thank you for the pep talks, reality checks, insightful wisdom, support and love. You've helped me grow so much as a person and I am extremely grateful to have you in my life.

To Alex for your candour, consistency, making me an honouree Big Atom team member and above all your incredible friendship. You're one of my favourite people to eat (and drink!) with and you've become like family to me.

To Rollo. Your strength, optimism, advice, patience, humour and kindness allowed me to finish this book. Thank you for the use of your kitchen and tastebuds, especially for the unsuccessful experiment that was my vegan lasagne (and my apologies to Dom too!).

To all the amazing humans who have helped me with kind words, testing recipes, long walks, lending me a home, encouragement, honesty and keeping me grounded, sane and functioning. Tash H, Tash S and Hammie (my OG!), Maddy, Izzy, Nicky, Georgie and James, Georgiana, Gussie, KJ, Wilhelm, Hugh and Lucy, Jeff and Emily, Henry and Alex, Lucy B, Will and Livvy, Annabel and Will, Francesca, Steph, Jasmine, Ro, Charlie, Sophie G, Alex and Hannah. I feel so lucky to know each and every one of you.

To my clients – thank you for trusting me with your health and helping me to become a better nutritionist with your questions, stories and journeys, without which I could never have written this book.